T0215102

Communication

Communication
The Social Matrix of Psychiatry

Jurgen Ruesch and
Gregory Bateson

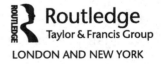

LONDON AND NEW YORK

Originally published in 1951 by W.W. Norton & Co, Inc.

Published 2008 by Transaction Publishers

Published 2017 by Routledge
2 Park Square, Milton Park, Abingdon, Oxon OX14 4RN
711 Third Avenue, New York, NY 10017, USA

Routledge is an imprint of the Taylor & Francis Group, an informa business

Copyright © 2008 by Taylor & Francis.

Notice:
Product or corporate names may be trademarks or registered trademarks, and are used only for identification and explanation without intent to infringe.

Library of Congress Catalog Number: 2008021778

Library of Congress Cataloging-in-Publication

Ruesch, Jurgen, 1909-
  Communication : the social matrix of psychiatry / Jurgen Ruesch and
Gregory Bateson.
      p. ; cm.
  Reprint. Originally published: New York : Norton, c1987.
  Includes bibliographical references and index.
  ISBN 978-1-4128-0614-5 (alk. paper)
      1. Communication in psychiatry. 2. Communication—Psychological
  aspects. 3. Social psychology. I. Bateson, Gregory, 1904-1980. II. Title.
  [DNLM: 1. Communication. 2. Psychiatry. 3. Social Environment. WM
  62 R921c 1987a]

RC437.2.R84 2008
616.89—dc22

                                                                    2008021778

ISBN 13: 978-1-4128-0614-5 (pbk)

CONTENTS

CONTENTS

PREFACE TO THE 1968 EDITION

THE INFORMATION sciences—perhaps the most exciting scientific and intellectual innovation of the twentieth century—emerged after World War II. The transactions of the early Macy Conferences on Cybernetics, Wiener's *Cybernetics: or Control and Communication in the Animal and the Machine* (1948), and Shannon and Weaver's *The Mathematical Theory of Communication* (1949) mark the beginnings of the new era. While the scientific community was trying to absorb the new ways of thinking that the communication engineers had introduced, the social structure of the universities underwent remarkable transformations. Professionals of various backgrounds began to collaborate in teams. The traditional separation of academic departments became blurred, and on the basis of interdisciplinary staffing new and more ambitious tasks were undertaken.

At about the same time, new orientations emerged in the field of mental health. Prior to the advent of tranquillizers, the main therapeutic effort of the psychiatrist was directed at the treatment and care of the major psychoses, and his principal tools were insulin and electroshock therapy. Then came World War II, and the psychiatrist was suddenly charged with the care of thousands of casualties who had suffered some form of psychological or social stress. Under these conditions, classical psychopathology proved to be ineffective for the understanding of personality disorders, psychoneuroses, and psychosomatic conditions. Instead, the formulations of dynamic psychiatry with their emphasis upon intra-psychic processes became more popular. However, psychoanalytic treatment methods proved to be too time-consuming, and line officers, flight surgeons, crew managers, and psychiatrists were hard-pressed to return men to active duty. New methods had to be developed, and attention converged on the fact that the group was of great help in the rehabilitation of neuropsychiatric casualties. Group procedures began to be part of the psychiatrist's resources.

At the time this book was written, it became abundantly clear that the age of the individual had passed. In spite of the temporary flowering of psychoanalysis, the main stream of events was no longer concerned with the private problems of people. The threat of atomic destruction, the mushrooming of the mass population, the horrifying specter of future famine, the progressive pollution of air and water, and the gradual decay of urban centers all pointed to the fact that the old ways of coping with human problems had become ineffective. Psychological man was dead and social man had taken his place. However, no unified or general theory was available at that time that could adequately represent the person, the group and society all within one system. True, there were theories pertaining to small groups on the one hand and to the societal order on the other; but what was lacking was a connecting link that would enable scientists to connect person to person, person to group, and group to the wider social order.

At this point the theoretical developments in the field of cybernetics and communication engineering were able to bridge the gap. By focusing not upon the person or the group, but upon the message and the circuit as units of study, a way was found to connect various entities. Notably in human systems the circuit which must be studied usually includes at least two persons. Indeed, the message must often be traced from its origin, as it passes from person to person through groups and machines, undergoing transformation, until it eventually reaches its intended destination, where its effects commonly act back upon the original source. The description of a theory of communication, adapted to the human situation, and particularly to the needs of psychiatry, was the end to which this book was originally written.

Nearly twenty years have elapsed since this volume was conceived, and in the meantime science has accelerated at an exponential rate. The convergence of physiology, ecology, and ethology—fields that study the organism's transactions with his physical and social environment—have resulted in the emergence of general systems theories of the biological sciences. The convergence of psychiatry, psychology, sociology, and anthropology—fields that study man's behavior alone and in groups— has led to what is now known as behavioral science. The convergence of administration, social organization, group management, and group therapy—fields that share in common the tendency to steer, organize, or change social behavior—have resulted in a theoretical body of knowledge concerned with social operations. Parallel to these scientific developments, we witness in the political arena an involvement of government in the heretofore more private domains of education, medical care, housing, and civil rights, with the result that the long-neglected social perspective of man's existence has achieved near parity with the technological views.

The evolution of communication has resulted not only in the development of better communication machinery but in a whole set of new types of human behavior. The computer, for one, has assumed the position of man's auxiliary brain, and the tasks of information storage, information retrieval, data scanning, computation, and translation no longer need be carried out by the human brain. Furthermore, computers can be used as scientific models of organisms or societies, and simulation of natural phenomena allows the scientist to check the correctness of his formulations. In the field of psychiatry, we have programs that are capable of simulating the behavior of patients and the behavior of psychiatrists. The conversation between two computers—one simulating the doctor and the other the patient—is almost indistinguishable from an interaction in the flesh. Computerized teaching programs and therapy machines are already well beyond the experimental stage. While in the past man interacted with animals or with people, he now has to face in addition autonomous quasi-organisms made of metal. Thus modern man has to contend with human interaction, man-machine interaction, and machine-machine interaction.

Communication thus has become the social matrix of modern life. In spite of the fact that the present book could describe neither the speed of technical developments nor the extent of the modern social commitments, it anticipated correctly the trend of future events—to wit, that the increasingly greater role of the mass media, the computers, and the self-steering devices in our civilization could be paralleled by a growing theoretical and practical emphasis upon social communication and social organization. Already twenty years ago it was clear that the complex machine cannot exist without its handmaiden, the social organization. The approach outlined in this volume also was to have a significant influence upon the later development of general systems theory and on the views prevailing in what is now called "social psychiatry."

After completion of this volume, both authors developed their ideas further. Gregory Bateson refined his theories of play, human interaction, and the ways of communication of schizophrenics, while Jurgen Ruesch sharpened his notions of nonverbal, disturbed, and therapeutic communication. The present edition of this volume, then, is intended to familiarize the reader with the foundations upon which these later developments were built.

THE AUTHORS

October, 1967

Communication

1 · VALUES, COMMUNICATION, AND CULTURE: An Introduction

By Jurgen Ruesch

TODAY, in the middle of the twentieth century, scientists and clinicians alike strive for mutual understanding. To renounce dogmatic views and to abandon scientific isolation is the fashion of our time. Psychiatrists have moved out of the enclosing walls of mental institutions and have found a new field of activity in the general hospitals of the community and in private practice. The transformation of the former alienist into a modern therapist and the change from static to dynamic principles necessitated a revision of psychiatric theories. While, in the past, theories of personality were concerned with one single individual, modern psychiatrists have come to the realization that such theories are of little use, because it is necessary to see the individual in the context of a social situation. Our technical civilization has reduced the intellectual isolation of people to a minimum, and modern means of communication and transportation accelerate the dissemination of information to such an extent that in the not too distant future we can expect that no individual or group will be able to escape such influences for long.

The authors have attempted in this book, which is dedicated to a presentation of the broader aspects of communication, to conceptualize interpersonal and psychotherapeutic events by considering the individual within the framework of a social situation. Focusing upon the larger societal systems, of which both psychiatrist and patient are an integral part, necessitated the development of concepts which would encompass large-scale events as well as happenings of an individual nature. We have sketched this relationship in a unified theory of communication, which would encompass events which link individual to individual, events which link the individual to the group, and ultimately, events of world-wide concern.

In the course of our investigation we had to examine the position of psychiatry within the framework of social science. Special attention was paid to the management of scientific information about the behavior of people and the interrelation of data obtained at the individual, group, and societal levels. We refer particularly to the dialectical difficulties which develop when the scientist operates at different levels of abstraction. To facilitate the consideration of an event, first within the narrower context of an individual organism, and then within the framework of a larger societal system, the concept of the social matrix was used. The term "social matrix," then, refers to a larger scientific system, of which both the psychiatrist and the patient are integral parts. This larger system, however, is of no immediate concern to the psychiatrist or to the patient at the time of interaction. Devoting attention to a particular subject matter, and delineating a circumscribed set of events, the limited concerns of the doctor-patient teams may not immediately affect the larger universe. Nonetheless, the smaller system is a part of the larger system; and conclusions drawn within this smaller system may become inaccurate or even invalid when seen in the framework of the wider over-all system.

This phenomenon we have related to the more general problem of "part and whole" (151). The physician and the psychiatrist, in their work, repeatedly deal with relationships between one cell and the surrounding tissue; one organ within an organism; an individual within the family group; a family within the community; and ultimately, perhaps, the community within the framework of the nation, and the nation within the United Nations. These varied foci of interest are usually watched and studied by different disciplines, all using their own concepts and their separate technical languages. Such divisions, though useful at one stage, can become merely obstructions at a later stage.

Therefore, in order to facilitate progress, we propose to use one single system for the understanding of the multiple aspects of human behavior. As of today, we believe that communication is the only scientific model which enables us to explain physical, intrapersonal, interpersonal, and cultural aspects of events within one system. By the use of one single system we eliminate the multiplicity of single universes, the multifarious vocabularies, and the controversies which arise because we, the scientists and clinicians, cannot understand each other. To introduce the reader to such a system of explanation in its application to the field of psychiatry the present volume has been written.

At this time the reader may ask what, if any, relationship exists between communication and the variety of topics which are presented in this volume. In reply we ask him to bear with us for a little while until such time as we have been able to demonstrate how value theory, psychiatric thinking, and observations about the American culture are intimately connected. We hope to show that these multifarious features which are included under the heading of social matrix are the silent determinants of our means of communication, and that communication is the link which connects psychiatry with all other sciences. It is well to remember that almost all phenomena included under the traditional heading of psychopathology are disturbances of communication and that such disturbances are in part defined by the culture in which they occur. Contemporary psychiatric theories were imported from Europe by Europeans, and inasmuch as psychiatric theories are implicitly theories of communication, they must undergo modification and progressive change when transplanted from one country to another. Therefore, considerable time and space have here been devoted to an understanding of the American system of communication and its implicit influence upon psychiatric practices and thinking.

At first sight, problems of communication seem to be of only secondary interest to the student of individual behavior. People act on their own, they do things alone, and at times they manage, exploit, coerce, or kill others without announcing their intention of doing so. But communication does not refer to verbal, explicit, and intentional transmission of messages alone; as used in our sense, the concept of communication would include all those processes by which people influence one another. The reader will recognize that this definition is based upon the premise that all actions and events have communicative aspects, as soon as they are perceived by a human being; it implies, furthermore, that such perception changes the information which an individual possesses and therefore influences him. In a social situation, where several people interact, things are even more complicated.

When persons convene, things happen. People have their feelings and thoughts, and both while they are together and afterwards, they act and react to one another. They themselves perceive their own actions, and other people who are present can likewise observe what takes place. Sensory impressions received and actions undertaken are registered; they leave some traces within the organism, and as a result of such experiences people's views of themselves and of each other may be confirmed, altered, or radically modified. The sum total of such traces, accumulated through the years by thousands of experiences, forms a person's character and determines in part the manner in which future events will be managed. The impressions received from the surroundings, from others, and from the self, as well as the retention of these impressions for future reference, can all be considered as being integral parts of a person's communication system. Inasmuch as a person's way of responding to perceived events necessitates the forwarding of messages to the peripheral effector organs, the intra-organismic network is conveniently considered as a part of the larger interpersonal, or even superpersonal (cultural) network.

What, then, the reader may ask, is not communication? In order to answer this problem, we must investigate the questions which a scientist wishes to answer. Where the relatedness of entities is considered, we deal with problems of communication; when entities are considered in isolation from one another, problems of communication are not relevant. To be interested in communication therefore becomes synonymous with assuming a definite scientific position with a viewpoint and interests focusing upon human relations. However, the scientific investigation of communication is made difficult by the fact that we have to communicate in order to investigate communication. Inasmuch as it is impossible to fix at any one moment our position as observers, we are never quite sure of that which we purport to observe. We can never abstain from communicating, and as human beings and members of a society, we are biologically compelled to communicate. Our sense organs are constantly on the alert and are registering the signals received, and inasmuch as our effector organs are never at rest, we are, at the same time, continually transmitting messages to the outside world. Therefore, our biological need to receive and transmit messages is in some ways a handicap to the investigation of the scientific processes of communication. In order to overcome this difficulty, it is necessary for us to make a structural assumption regarding the state of signs and signals within our own organism. This end result of perception and transmission we refer to as information.

The acquisition and retention of information is paramount in any system of communication. In order to retain some traces of messages received and sent, and in order to evaluate these, the human organism is equipped to detect common features in apparently diverse events. The elements or patterns which are common to a variety of happenings are of necessity abstract, and it is these abstract relationships which are retained by the organism. However, in order to proceed with abstraction, the organism must be exposed to a sufficient number of events which contain the same factors. Only then is a person equipped to cope with the most frequent happenings that he may encounter. If a person is able to predict events, and if he possesses the ability to cope with certain happenings, he is said to have relevant information. As far as we know, that which is referred to as information consists of an arrangement of nervous impulses and connections. This arrangement must consist of relationships which are systematically derived from those among the original events outside the organism.

In the social sphere, the acquisition of information about relatedness to people occurs through continuity and consistency of exposure to similar social events; it begins with the child's experiences with his mother, then with members of his family, and later with contemporaries at school and on the playground.

The youngster learns from adults and from his age mates to follow rules and to master the obstacles which he encounters. The repetitive character of social events teaches people to react in stereotyped ways; and stereotyped behavior creates, of course, stereotyped surroundings. Therefore, when we speak of a social matrix, in which interpersonal events take place, we refer to the repetitive and consistent bombardments with stimuli to which human beings are exposed. These originate, on the one hand, in the social behavior of other people and, on the other hand, in the objects, plants, and animals with which people surround themselves. Gradually the stimuli perceived and the responses chosen become stylized; the stimulus shapes the response, and once the response has been learned, the individual is conditioned to seek those stimuli which will elicit his learned responses. This whole process can be compared to the bed which a river cuts into the surface of the earth. The channel is formed by the water, but the river banks also control the direction of flow, so that a system of interaction is established in which cause and effect can no longer be isolated. Stimulus and response are thus welded into a unit; this unit we shall refer to as "value."

Values are therefore, so to speak, simply preferred channels of communication or relatedness. Information about the values which people hold enables us to interpret their messages and to influence their behavior. Values are not only characteristic of an individual but are also held by groups of people and by whole cultures. The reader will recognize that as soon as interpretation of messages is considered, no clear distinction can be made between communication theory, value theory, and anthropological statements about culture. This combination of features is the medium in which we all operate; therefore we refer to it as the social matrix.

As individuals we are usually not fully aware of the existence of this social matrix. Unable fully to encompass the effects of our own actions upon others, and because of our limited human perspective, we are unlikely to grasp the magnitude and nature of what happens. When we quarrel with a family member, or when we attempt to explain the reasons for a rise in the price of butter, we tend to treat such incidents as unique; thus, unaware that thousands of other people might have similar experiences, we blame our relatives or we curse the grocer. As a matter of fact our behavior in such situations is already both a response to other people's reactions and a stimulus for their behavior. Our personal and interpersonal concerns, the immediate foci of our daily life, make it difficult for us to appreciate fully the wider aspects of social events. Therefore, in this book, we have made it our task to illustrate some of the relations which exist between individual, group, and culture. While for the average person it is quite sufficient to possess some practical working knowledge of these matters, the psychiatrist, in addition, must possess explicit and systematic knowledge of these relationships if he wishes to help his patients. The relationship between superpersonal systems on the one hand, and interpersonal and individual systems on the other, is not merely a dialectic fancy of the scientist, but is embedded in the daily needs of the individual, whose life and sanity require that he be able to communicate successfully with other human beings. To the achievement of this end the psychiatrist has dedicated his life.

After introducing our subject matter to the reader it might be worth while to say a word about the *methods* we used to study the social matrix. It is well to remember that regardless of whether the scientist studies psychiatric, social, or cultural phenomena, sooner or later he has to consider the individual. The only thing that differs is the data obtained from individuals. Therefore in carrying out this study we have found it convenient and necessary to keep clear in our thinking the differences between the various sorts of data with which we have had to deal. Especially is this true of the differences between participant experience and experimental operation, and between observation of behavioral acts and introspective reports. The fact must be faced that when a culture or subculture is studied as an integrated communication system, it is necessary to consider in the scheme of scientific operations the following circumstances:

(a) That the members of the population studied make generalizations about their own culture.

(b) That the investigator observes interaction and communication between the members of the population as a neutral spectator.

(c) That each member of the population has his own view of his own roles and can in some measure report these to the observer.

(d) Lastly, that the investigator obtains important insight from his own personal interaction with members of the population.

Each of these circumstances determines a particular way of collecting data, and it is necessary to insist that the data collected in any one of these ways are not the same, either in their order of abstraction or in the distortions which they introduce, as the data collected in one of the other ways. In general, it may be said that these four types of data are mutually corrective and that an undue specialization in any one of the four leads to a distorted picture. The sorts of distortion which result from over-specialization in each type of data collecting may here be mentioned:

If the investigator overspecializes in his attention to what people say about their own culture, he will arrive at an idealized or stereotyped picture of that culture; he will collect a system of social generalizations which ignore the actual behavior of actual people. His picture will be a function of the culture which he is studying, because he will collect stereotypes which are themselves culturally determined; but it will be a distorted function. Further, if the investigator is sociologically minded, he may be guilty of the sort of oversimplification which occurs in organizational charts, forgetting the human individuals and seeing only their defined functions.

Similarly, if the investigator specializes in being a neutral observer of interaction between members of a population, he may build up a picture of customs and character types from which human individuality and the idiosyncrasies of motivation will be lacking. He might, for example, arrive at the position common in anthropology of paying attention to individual behavior, only to use his observations of people's reactions to point up their culturally stylized attitudes.

If, on the other hand, the investigator specializes in collecting personal introspective reports, he will arrive at the distortions characteristic of the overspecialized therapist; he may see the individuals as isolated entities, not related to each other or to himself. He will be limited to a discussion of their internal structure and dynamics, not seeing the structure and dynamisms of the larger social whole.

Finally, the scientist who overspecializes in participant experience will perceive individual trends and interaction but will tend to ignore the more static phenomena of convention, social organization, and other social determinants. His picture will resemble one which might be drawn by an overspecialized psychiatrist who sees the unique dynamics and flux of an individual's responses to himself without seeing that individual's life as socially determined.

Also, it is of interest to note that the systematic differences and distortions which follow when the investigator takes a particular view of the system which he is studying, or when he specializes in a particular method of collecting data, are themselves clues to his value system. The nature or slant of his knowledge is determined by his methods of obtaining that knowledge and by his notions of what knowledge is. If we describe his selective awareness—his structuring of perception—we shall, in fact, be describing his system of values.

As authors, we are fully aware that whatever we may say about value systems of psychiatrists, patients, or the American culture will be colored by our own personal values. On the other hand, we are also fully aware that no scientific observer can escape being bound to his subjective way of perceiving, inasmuch as any investigator is an integral part of the communication system in which he and the observed—be it human, animal, or object—participate. In the present study this danger of distortion has been acknowledged by including various types of data and by having more than one author, each with a different background and viewpoint, participate in the evaluation of the data. This combination of contrasting types of data and differently trained observers tends to minimize the distortions mentioned above.

The facts, combinations, and concepts presented in this volume are based upon the following experiences of the authors:

(a) We have studied psychiatrists [1] in non-controlled interviews in their homes, their offices, our offices, or wherever the opportunity presented itself. In this type of interview the focus of the investigation centered in the interaction with the psychiatrists, in order to gain a better picture of the informant's interpersonal approaches.

(b) In addition to these innumerable interviews in informal settings, about thirty sessions of one or two hours' duration with more than thirty different psychiatrists were recorded on wire with the knowledge of all participants. These interviews were not shaped according to questionnaires, nor were the psychiatrists subjected to detailed questioning such as must be resorted to in linguistic or genealogical studies. The approach was sometimes that in which an anthropologist gives freedom to his informant to follow the lines of his own thought guided only by occasional questions and suggestions of topic, and sometimes that in which the interviewer expresses his own honest opinions, leading to argument and discussion. The open-ended suggestion of a topic tended to focus the conversation upon the psychiatrist's therapeutic interest, and eventually led to his individualistic formulations, which tended to reveal more clearly the value system which governed his therapeutic operations.

(c) We have attended psychiatric meetings in which either theoretical issues were discussed or cases were presented, and we have studied the way psychiatrists relate themselves to each other and the way they talk about theory and about patients.

(d) We have as patients participated in individual therapy and experienced the psychiatrist in his function as therapist.

(e) We have examined the literature of American psychiatry and the assumptions contained therein. The printed sources which we studied were confined to the contemporary publications of leading psychiatrists, psychoanalysts, and psychotherapists of every school of thought. European sources were not par-

[1] This work was part of a research study on nonverbal communication in psychotherapy, which is in part supported by a research grant from the Division of Mental Hygiene, U. S. Public Health Service. In particular, this grant enabled us to do the work mentioned in paragraphs (a), (b), and (g) above.

ticularly emphasized because they do not reflect American thinking on the subject.

(f) We have studied the popular stereotypes of the psychiatrist as they appear in cartoons and anecdotes as well as the formal and informal reactions of the public to psychiatry.

(g) We have recorded many hundreds of hours of therapeutic sessions. Several therapist-patient teams were followed longitudinally and many more teams were studied cross-sectionally. These recorded interviews were then analyzed by the authors for material pertinent to the value systems of both therapist and patient, and especially for the study of the modification of values in and during therapy (135), (136), (142), (146), (148), (150).

(h) We have made a study of the American cultural milieu in which the psychiatrist operates (139), (140), (143). The value premises of the American culture were derived from sources listed in the bibliography, from years of interaction of the authors with Americans, and from the study of the systems and methods of communication in press, movies, radio, advertising, courts, hospitals, and other institutions. In brief, our impressions, derived from living in America, have been drawn on and checked by discussions between the authors and by current observations during the progress of the study.

Psychiatry and anthropology are still at the stage of being descriptive sciences; and because, in such sciences, the theoretical premises are left implicit, these sciences have difficulty in accumulating a coherent body of clearly formulated hypotheses. The present book has been dedicated to the task of stating and illustrating at length the premises which underlie the various approaches to social science. We have chosen psychiatry as the focus of our attention because the psychiatrist in his daily practice is concerned with disturbances of communication; he and the communication engineer, of all scientists, seem to be most aware of the laws of communication. The essence of our message to the reader is that communication is the matrix in which all human activities are embedded. In practice, communication links object to person and person to person; and scientifically speaking, this interrelatedness is understood best in terms of systems of communication.

In gathering information relevant to communication we had to combine the most diversified approaches. In this book the reader will encounter a number of chapters which have been labeled in succession as interdisciplinary, psychiatric, psychological, integrative, anthropological, philosophical, and epistemological approaches. In so naming the chapters we have attempted on the one hand to define the position and viewpoints of the observer, and on the other hand, to show that in spite of different viewpoints, such observers use a system of communication common to all. Furthermore, the chapters have been arranged in such a way as to present a progression from the more common observations of a concrete nature to the more abstract and theoretical formulations. The use of a variety of topics, of differences in approach, and of multiple levels of abstraction was thought to encompass the field of human communication more thoroughly than would have been possible by any single approach. Hence psychiatric, psychological, and anthropological concepts have been synthesized with theories derived from cybernetics and communication engineering.

The present volume is concerned with theoretical matters. The notions of information, communication, preference, and value are notoriously obscure, and the phenomena associated with these notions are exceedingly difficult to dissect. This book is concerned with such dissection. It is a descriptive, not an experimental, study, and this fact has curious implications:

In an ideal experimental presentation, a hypothesis is stated, the outcome of a crucial experiment is described, and at the end, it is clear what contribution has been made to theoretical knowledge; the hypothesis is fortified, modified, or discarded. In a descriptive study things are not so simple because the theoretical premises of the scientist determine his techniques of description and have themselves been determined in part by his experience of the phenomena which he is describing. At the end of such a presentation, it may be clear that certain new facts have been added to knowledge, but it is usually very unclear what contribution has been made at a more theoretical level.

Although each of the two authors is individually responsible for the chapters he has written, in thought and context the book is the result of interdisciplinary teamwork between a psychiatrist and an anthropologist. Data related to the uniqueness of the individual are therefore combined with data related to the more abstract similarities which men have in common. We invite the reader to participate in judging whether or not communication is the common denominator which bridges the gap between the various fields of social science. If the answer is in the affirmative, the first step has been made towards the establishment of a more unified theory of human behavior.

BASIC PREMISES

To help the reader to understand our viewpoint and to fixate the point of departure of our sometimes rather theoretical considerations, we have verbalized our basic premises in a few sentences. These may serve as milestones for that which we shall illustrate, amplify, and pursue further in the later chapters of our book.

Delineation of Universe: The unit of consideration is the social situation.

Social Situation: A social situation is established when people enter into interpersonal communication.

Interpersonal Communication: An interpersonal event is characterized by:

(a) The presence of expressive acts on the part of one or more persons.
(b) The conscious or unconscious perception of such expressive actions by other persons.
(c) The return observation that such expressive actions were perceived by others. The perception of having been perceived is a fact which deeply influences and changes human behavior.

Intrapersonal Communication: The consideration of intrapersonal events becomes a special case of interpersonal communication. An imaginary entity made up of condensed traces of past experiences represents *within* an individual the missing outside person. However, a crucial difference exists between interpersonal and intrapersonal communication with regard to the registration of mistakes. In the interpersonal situation the effects of purposive or expressive actions can be evaluated and if necessary corrected. In intrapersonal or fantasy communication, to perceive that one misinterprets one's own messages is extremely difficult, if not impossible, and correction rarely, if ever, occurs.

Mass Communication: A social event may be characterized by mass communication—e.g., through the media of radio, television, movies, and the press. When exposed to such mass communications, an individual is likely to feel on the one hand, that he is a participant in a larger superpersonal system, and on the other hand, that he is unable to delineate the system. This contradiction is brought about by the fact that in mass communications the originators and recipients of messages are so numerous that they usually remain anonymous. Therefore, under such conditions, the individual is not able to observe the effect of his own messages upon others, nor can he communicate his personal reactions to a message originating from committees, organizations, or institutions. Cause and effect become blurred, correction and self-correction of messages become delayed in time and removed in space; if correction finally occurs, it often is no longer appropriate.

Communication Apparatus: The communication apparatus of man has to be viewed as a functional entity without anatomical localization. The reader should be reminded that several parallel sets of expressions exist to denote the phenomena of communication. While the engineer's "communication center" corresponds to the mentalist's "psyche," the organicist refers to it as "central nervous system." We believe that one of the most important changes which must follow from interchange of theories between engineers and psychiatrists is an increasing precision in the use of mentalist phrasings. Engineers and physiologists are still very far from giving us an organic base on which mentalist theories can be built, but they have already given us certain general notions about the characteristics of networks of relays, and these general notions must guide and restrict our loose use of mentalist abstractions. In our view, the communication apparatus of man is composed of:

(a) his sense organs, the receivers
(b) his effector organs, the senders
(c) his communication center, the place of origin and destination of all messages
(d) the remaining parts of the body, the shelter of the communication machinery.

Limitations of Communication: The limitations of man's communications are determined by the capacity of his intrapersonal network, the selectivity of his receivers, and the skill of his effector organs. The number of incoming and outgoing signals, as well as the signals that can be transmitted within the organism, is limited. Beyond a certain maximum any increase in number of messages in transit leads to a jamming of the network, and so to a decrease in the number of messages which reach their appropriate destinations. This type of disruption of the communication system the psychiatrist calls anxiety. It is subject to conjecture whether reduction of the number of incoming messages, and messages in transit below a certain minimum, may lead to a "starvation phenomenon." From information gathered in the study of infants it seems that mental retardation is the result of insufficient interaction with others. There is also a more obscure limitation of communication which results from the difficulty of discussing the basic premises and codification of a system of signals in those same signals. This difficulty is shown to be of special relevance in the psychiatric situation, where the patient and therapist have to achieve communication about their own understanding of their own utterances. The same difficulty is also present in all attempts to communicate between persons of different cultural backgrounds.

Function of Communication: Man uses his communication system:

(a) to receive and transmit messages and to retain information;
(b) to perform operations with the existing information for the purpose of deriving new conclusions which were not directly perceived and for reconstructing past and anticipating future events;

(c) to initiate and modify physiological processes within his body;

(d) to influence and direct other people and external events.

Effect of Communication: Communication facilitates specialization, differentiation, and maturation of the individual. In the process of maturation reliance upon protective and corrective actions of others is gradually replaced by interdependence upon contemporaries in terms of communication. Instead of looking to elders for guidance, the adult person seeks information from contemporaries on how best to solve a problem. Exchange is substituted for receiving, and action of self replaces actions of others.

Interference and Communication: Interference with goal-directed behavior of an individual gives rise to the alarm reaction. If the interference can be successfully disposed of or avoided altogether, the alarm reaction will recede. However, frequently the source of interference cannot be avoided or eliminated. Under such circumstances, the sharing of anxiety with non-anxious or non-threatening individuals by means of communication becomes an efficient device for tolerating the impact of interference.

Adjustment: Successful communication with self and with others implies correction by others as well as self-correction. In such a continuing process, up-to-date information about the self, the world, and the relationship of the self to the world leads to the acquisition of appropriate techniques, and eventually increases the individual's chances of mastery of life. Successful communication therefore becomes synonymous with adaptation and life.

Disturbances of Communication: Abnormalities of behavior are described in terms of disturbances of communication. In the past, these disturbances have been summarized under the heading of psychopathology. It is well to remember that the term "organic" refers to disruption of the internal communication machinery, that "intrapersonal" refers to a network limited to one individual, and that "interpersonal" refers to a network composed of several individuals. Complete descriptions of disturbances of communication therefore include:

(a) on a technical level, statements about the communication apparatus, the dimensions of the network, and the functional implications as well as physical aspects of transmission and reception.

(b) on a semantic level, statements about the accuracy with which a series of symbols transmit the desired meaning of a message, including semantic distortions.

(c) on an interaction level, statements about the effectiveness of the transmission of information upon the behavior of people in an attempt to achieve a desired effect.

Psychiatric Therapy: Psychiatric therapy aims at improving the communication system of the patient. The neurophysiologist, neurologist, and neurosurgeon endeavor to improve the internal communication apparatus of the patient on a technical level, while the psychotherapist aims at restoring a broken-down system of interpersonal communication on a semantic or interaction level. This is achieved either by reducing the number of incoming messages and preventing jamming, or by increasing the number of messages in transit and preventing isolation and starvation. Once communication of the patient with the self and with others has improved, correction and self-correction of information provide the foundations for a change in the conduct of the patient.

Nature of Psychotherapy: Regardless of the school of thought adhered to, or the technical terms used, the therapist's operations always occur in a social context. Implicitly, therefore, all therapists use communication as a method of influencing the patient. The differences that exist between the therapist and the patient are differences in their systems of value, which can be traced to differences in the codification or evaluation of perceived events.

The Psychiatrist's Value System: In order to understand the differences which exist between the communication system of the patient and that of his fellow-man, the psychiatrist must possess information about both. If the psychiatrist's communication system were similar to that of the patient, he would be unable to help him; if the psychiatrist's communication system is identical with that of the people surrounding the patient, he will notice that the patient is different, but still will be unable to help him. Therefore, it becomes necessary for the psychiatrist to possess values which are somewhat different from those of the patient and somewhat different from those of the core group.

The Psychiatrist and Culture Change: The differences in the psychiatrist's value system from those of the core group arise from specific life experiences. Essentially they are related to experiences of culture contact and repeated exposure to differing systems of value during the formative years. Such conditions sharpen the social perception of the future psychiatrist and make him aware of the fact that values differ from group to group. Being forced to reinterpret his own position whenever he meets a new group, he develops the necessary means which enable him to perceive and evaluate the various communication systems of other people. Such basic life experiences are necessary if a man wishes to become a successful therapist. Training merely supplies a system for an orderly arrangement of these basic life experiences.

Distorted Communication and Marginal Status of Patients: The values which distinguish patients from other people and from the therapist are a result of the particular social situations in which the patients were reared. Unable to assimilate divergent trends within the home, or between home and surroundings, these patients have never developed satisfactory means of communication. This results in marginal status as compared to the people who make up the core of the group in which the patient lives.

Mental Hygiene: The psychiatrist's work is aimed at helping the patient to acquire a communication system which is similar to that of the core group; and as an interpreter, he familiarizes the core group with the peculiarities of marginal man. The nature of the mental hygiene movement and other endeavors is to prevent the development of disturbances of communication which, in turn, are directly or indirectly responsible for disturbances of behavior.

2 · COMMUNICATION AND HUMAN RELATIONS: An Interdisciplinary Approach

By Jurgen Ruesch

THE FIELD of communication is concerned with human relatedness. Every person, plant, animal, and object emits signals which, when perceived, convey a message to the receiver. This message changes the information of the receiver and hence may alter his behavior. Change in behavior of the receiver, in turn, may or may not perceptibly influence the sender. Sometimes the effect of a message is immediate; at other times the message and its effect are so far apart in time and space that the observer fails to connect the two events. For purposes of our presentation however, we shall be concerned more with the immediate effects of messages and their influence upon the behavior of people.

CHANNELS OF COMMUNICATION IN EVERYDAY LIFE

In order to familiarize the reader with the varieties of human communication, let us view the experiences of Mr. A as he proceeds with his daily activities. In the morning when Mr. A enters his office he reads his incoming mail (written communication). In sorting his mail he encounters a number of pamphlets which are designed to describe the merits of various business machines (pictorial communication). Through the open window the faint noise of a radio is heard, as the voice of an announcer clearly praises the quality of a brand of toothpaste (spoken com-

21

munication). When his secretary enters the room she gives him a cheerful "good morning," which he acknowledges with a friendly nod of his head (gestural communication) while he continues with his conversation on the telephone (spoken communication) with a business associate. Later in the morning he dictates a number of letters to his secretary, then he holds a committee meeting (group communication), where he gathers the advice of his associates. In this meeting a number of new governmental regulations (mass communication) and their effect upon the policies of the firm are discussed. Later in the meeting a resolution to the employees of the firm concerning the annual bonus (mass and group communication) is considered. After the committee has adjourned, Mr. A, engaged in thoughts concerning unfinished business (communication with self), slowly crosses the street to his restaurant for lunch. On the way he sees his friend Mr. B, who in a great hurry enters the same luncheon place (communication through action), and Mr. A decides to sit by himself rather than to join his friend, who will probably gulp down his coffee and hurry on (communication with self). While waiting, Mr. A studies the menu (communication through printed word) but the odor of a juicy steak deflects his gaze (chemical communication); it is so appetizing that he orders one himself. After lunch he decides to buy a pair of gloves. He enters a men's store and with the tips of his fingers carefully examines the various qualities of leather (communication through touch). After leisurely concluding the purchase, he decides to take the afternoon off and to escort his son on a promised trip to the zoo. On the way there, John, watching his father drive through the streets, asks him why he always stops at a red light and why he does not stop at a green light (communication by visual symbol). As they approach the zoo, an ambulance screams down the street, and Mr. A pulls over to the side of the road and stops (communication by sound). As they sit there he explains to his son that the church across the street is the oldest in the state, built many years ago, and still standing as a landmark in the community (communication through material culture). After paying admission to the zoo (communication through action), they leisurely stroll over to visit the elephants. Here John laughs at the antics of an elephant who sprays water through his trunk at one of the spectators (communication through action), sending him into near flight. Later on in the afternoon Mr. A yields to the pressure of his son, and they enter a movie house to see a cartoon (communication through pictures). Arriving home, Mr. A dresses in order to attend a formal dinner and theater performance (communication through the arts).

These examples may suffice to illustrate the varieties of social situations in which communication occurs. Let us next consider how a scientist can conceptualize these various events in a more systematized fashion.

THE CONTEXT IN WHICH COMMUNICATION OCCURS

The scientific approach to communication has to occur on several levels of complexity. In a first step we shall be concerned with the definition of the context in which communication occurs. This context is summarized by the label which people give to specific social situations. Identification of a social situation is important both for the participant who wishes to communicate and for the scientist who aims at conceptualizing the processes of communication.

The Perception of the Perception

A social situation is established as soon as an exchange of communication takes place; and such exchange begins with the moment in which the actions of the other individual are perceived as responses—that is, as evoked by the sender's message and therefore as comments upon that message, giving the sender an opportunity of judging what the message meant to the receiver. Such communication about communication is no doubt difficult, because it is usually implicit rather than explicit, but it must be present if an exchange of messages is to take place. The perception of the perception, as we might call this phenomenon, is the sign that a silent agreement has been reached by the participants, to the effect that mutual influence is to be expected.

The mutual recognition of having entered into each other's field of perception equals the establishment of a system of communication. The criteria of mutual awareness of perception are in all cases instances of communications about communication. If a person "A" raises his voice to attract person "B's" attention, he is thereby making a statement about communication. He may, for example, be saying, "I am communicating with you," or he may be saying, "I am not listening to you; I am doing the talking"—and so on. Similarly, all punctuations of the stream of emitted signals are statements about how that stream is to be broken down into sections, and significantly all modifications of the stream of signals, which implicitly or explicitly assign roles either to the self or to the other, are statements about communication. If "A" adds the word "please" to a verbal request, he is making a statement about that request; he is giving instructions about the mood or role which he desires the listener to adopt when he interprets the verbal stream. He is adding a signal to cause a modification in the receiver's interpretation. In this sense the added signal is a communication about communication as well as a statement about the relationship between two persons.

The Position of the Observer within the System of Communication

Dependent upon whether an observer is a participant in a group discussion, or remains a scientific observer who, rather aloof and with a minimum of participation, proceeds to make scientific notes, the information about what happens is going to vary. The position of the observer, his viewpoints and foci of interest, his degree of participation, and his lucidity in interpreting rules, roles, and situations will determine that which he is going to report.

When a scientist endeavors to study such complicated matters as human relations, he conveniently divides the universe into segments small enough so that the events which occur within such a subdivision can be observed and recorded in a satisfactory manner. In proceeding from the larger to the smaller units of consideration, the scientist has to guard against pitfalls which may arise from his personal focus of endeavor, his personal views, and his particular perspectives. His position may be likened to that of a visitor to a museum of art, who never succeeds in seeing the front and back views of a statue at the same moment. From a position in back of the statue, for example, he will be unable to predict the facial expression until he has seen it from the front. To obtain a complete impression, he has to walk around the statue; and as he moves, a new perspective will open at every step until the combination of all impressions will enable the visitor to construct within himself a small-scale model of the marble figure. Matters get even more complicated if one considers that not all visitors go to the museum with the same purpose in mind. Some wish to obtain a quick impression of the treasures on hand; others want to undertake detailed studies in preparation for an artist's career; some want to meet people who have the same interests. Thus, varying with their purpose, any of several persons gathered around the statue might retain within himself a different view of the marble figure.

The scientist is very much in the same position as the spectator of the statue, with the exception that, to achieve a more complete understanding of what he is doing and of what happens in nature, he does not limit himself to perception and observation only. In order to satisfy his curiosity, he compensates for his human limitations of perception by creating a theory. In brief, he proceeds about as follows: First, he postulates that there are events. An event is defined as an occurrence which occupies a small part of the general four-dimensional, space-time continuum. If the scientist happens to observe such an event and if it can be verified by others, he refers to his statement of it as a fact. Sometimes he adds to his observations certain physical measurements: he makes observations on the relations between the event and his own measuring rod. In order to be able to measure or to experiment, however, the scientist needs a hypothesis; it is nothing but a provisional, tentative theory, a supposition that he adopts temporarily in order to add to the already well-established knowledge a series of new facts. Hypotheses thus guide all future research work. When a hypothesis—that is, an assumption without proof—can be substantiated by fact, it becomes a theory. The latter can be described as being the result of reasoning with the intent to derive from a body of known facts some general or abstract principles. Such principles can then be applied to other bodies of knowledge in order to finally interconnect the information about events in a larger time-space continuum. The scientist has to rely upon theory, because only few events are accessible to direct observation or measurement. The majority of processes in nature or within the human being himself are either so slow or so fast that they escape perception. Theory is then used to combine the known facts into a network, allowing for interpolation and extrapolation, reconstruction of past and prediction of future events.

At this point the reader will recognize that as soon as we talk or think about a social situation we have to define our own position as observers. Therefore, every individual becomes a scientific observer as soon as he engages in communication.

To evaluate daily events and to guide future actions, every single human being possesses a private scientific system. To students of human behavior, the private systems of others are accessible only in a rather restricted manner. That which is assimilated by the human being in terms of stimuli—be it food, oxygen, sound, or light—and that which the individual produces in heat, waste materials, or purposive action is accessible to investigation. Whatever happens between intake and output is known on a restricted scale only; through introspection and, in recent years, by means of X-rays and radioactive tracer substances, scientists have been able to follow some of the processes which take place within the organism. For practical purposes, however, events occurring in other persons are accessible to an observer in terms of inference alone; all he observes is the stimuli which reach the other person and the latter's reactions; the rest is subject to conjecture. Furthermore, the observer, being a social stimulus for others, possesses knowledge about the origin and the nature of some of the stimuli which he feeds to other individuals. In such a system, which includes the observer as an integral part, the actions of the first person are stimuli for the second person and the responses of the second person are stimuli for the first person.

Identification of Roles and Rules

Once the position of the observing reporter is clearly defined and a social situation has been established because people have entered into communication, it is left to the participants to identify the social situation. The label which a person is going to give to a social situation is intimately connected with the rules which govern the situation, as well as the roles which the various participants aɪ _ to assume. It is obvious that each person has his own views regarding the label of the situation and that much confusion results when people disagree as to what a situation is about. Through communication with others, roles are mutually assigned, and by means of mutual exploration agreement is frequently reached as to the nature of the situation. Used in connection with communication, the term "role" refers to nothing but the code which is used to interpret the flow of messages. For example, the statements of a person who wishes to sell an automobile are going to be interpreted in a sense quite different from that which they would have if the person were to make the same statements in the role of an automobile buyer. Awareness of a person's role in a social situation enables others to gauge correctly the meaning of his statements and actions.

Once the roles of the self and of all other participants have been established, the code for interpreting the conversation is given. The number of roles which people can assume is limited, and elsewhere we have calculated that their number is probably about twenty-five (see p. 405 in ref. 149). A mature individual is capable of mastering this number of roles in the course of a lifetime.

Any social situation is governed by explicit or implicit rules; these rules may be created on the spur of the moment for a particular situation, or they may be the result of centuries of tradition. In the context of communication, rules can be viewed as directives which govern the flow of messages from one person to another. Inasmuch as rules are usually restrictive, they limit the possibilities of communication between people, and above all, they restrict the actions of the participating persons. Rules can be viewed as devices which either stabilize or disrupt a given communication system, and they provide directives for all eventualities. The meaning of rules, regulations, and laws can be understood best if one thinks of a card game in which several persons participate: The channels of communication are prescribed, the sequence of messages is regulated, and the effects of messages are verifiable. The rules also explain that certain messages, at certain times, addressed to certain people, are not admissible, and that known penalties are imposed upon those who break the rules. Furthermore, regulations pertaining to the beginning of the game, the division of functions in terms of roles, and the termination of the game are always included (see p. 401 in ref. 149; see also ref. 168.)

The Label of the Social Situation

A social situation is established when people have entered into communication; the state of communication is determined by the fact that a person perceives that his perception has been noted by others. As soon as this fact has been established, a system of communication can be said to exist. At that point selective reception, purposive transmission, and corrective processes take place and the circular characteristics and self-corrective mechanisms of the system of communication become effective. This implies that roles have been assigned and rules established. The participants in a social situation experience these events more or less consciously, and the experience induces them to label a social situation. Such a label specifies not only the status assignment (roles) of the participants and the rules pertaining to the gathering, but also the task or the purpose to which a social situation is devoted. A funeral, for example, serves another purpose than a wedding, and communications vary accordingly. Elsewhere (see p. 398 in ref. 149) we have advanced the idea that the social situations encountered by the average person number less than forty, a figure which the normally gifted person can master easily.

In identifying social labels it is obvious that external criteria are extremely helpful. If people are dressed in mourning, and others know the significance of the special clothing, they will all agree as to the label of the situation, and communications are therefore limited and interpreted under the seal of the situation. Different and difficult is the situation, however, when two strangers meet—for example, in a western frontier setting, around 1850. External cues of behavior might not have helped them recognize each other's roles. One man, for example, might have been intent on murder, or persecution, or trade. In such cases the label has to be worked out as time goes on, and new rules created. The interval which elapses between the establishment of a social situation and its definite label may vary. Some persons are very skillful in bringing about a clarification of the situation; others, especially neurotics, may experience great anxiety until roles, rules, and purpose have been defined.

THE SIMPLER SYSTEMS OF COMMUNICATION

When a person is alone, the system of communication is confined to that one organism. If there are two people, then the communication network embraces both organisms. If there are many people, the network embraces the whole group, and if we consider many groups, we may talk about a cultural network. In a one-person communication system the signals travel along the established pathways of the body. In a two-or-more-person system the signals travel both along the pathways of the body and through the media which separate the bodies.

Let us now consider first the human instruments of communication and the bodily pathways used for communication. A man's organism as a whole can be conceived of as an instrument of communication, equipped with sense organs, the receivers; with effector organs, the senders; with internal transmitters, the humoral and nervous pathways; and with a center, the brain. However, the reader is warned not to think in anatomical terms when considering the internal network of communication; more appropriate is the comparison of the individual with a social organization. Within the organized confines of a state, for example, messages from the borders and from all parts of the nation are transmitted to the capital and to all other points by means of an intricate network. The messages can be conveyed by radio, telephone, telegraph, or word of mouth; printed messages may be carried by air, ship, rail, on wheels, on foot, or on horseback. The person that first reports an event usually does not engage in any extensive traveling to spread the news. Instead, through a system of relays the message is transmitted to other places and people. Each relay station may alter, amplify, condense, or abstract the original message for local use; and frequently after long transit any resemblances between the first and the last report are purely coincidental. This analogy applies well to the consideration of the human organism.

The sense organs, for example, are found scattered from head to toe on the external surface of the body and in or around internal organs as well. Sensitive to stimuli which originate in the surroundings as well as in the body itself, the end organs act as stations of impulse transformation. Regardless of whether the original stimulus consists of a series of light or sound waves or of a chemical reagent, the sense organs transform that which is perceived into impulses which are suitable for internal transmission within the organism. Likewise, it does not matter whether these impulses are conducted along afferent pathways from peripheral and cranial nerves to the brain or along humoral pathways, or perhaps contiguously from cell to cell within a given organ. The essence of the matter is that all living tissue is equipped with the ability to respond to the impact of specific stimuli; such responsiveness may be called irritability. The nature of this responsiveness is determined in part by the type of stimulus which is perceived and in part by the nature of the reacting tissues, organs, and systems of organs. For greater economy and efficiency the stimulus perceived on the surface of the body or within the organism itself is transformed in such a way that it can be transmitted properly; and likewise, the impulses originating in the brain and other regulatory centers are transformed in several stations before they reach the effector organs or, even more remotely, the sense organs of another person.

Our effector organs, the striped and smooth muscles of the body, react to stimuli originating in the organism itself. The irritability of the muscles, when stimulated, results in contractions which in turn may give rise to movements of the limbs, to motions of the body in space, to passage of air through the windpipe, and subsequently to sound or to internal movements of the intestinal tract or the circulatory system. Whenever activities of an organ or of the whole organism are perceived by the self or by others, they constitute communicative acts which warrant interpretation. The higher centers of the nervous systems and perhaps certain glands evaluate messages originating in single organs, and a person may respond automatically, sometimes not being consciously aware of this transmission. Such automatic responses are termed reflexes if the circuit, with the exception of the stimulus, is located entirely within one organism. In transmission of messages from person to person information pertaining to the state of the organism of the speakers is frequently transmitted without the awareness of the participants. In social situations, for example, people automatically evaluate the other person's attitude—that is, whether it is friendly or hostile. Without being conscious of their own responses they will be more cautious and alert when facing a hostile individual than when they encounter an apparently harmless person. More complex interpersonal messages, especially when coded in verbal form, require a more conscious evaluation and interpretation. But regardless of the complexity of the message or the extent of the network, the basic principles remain the same.

A neutral observer, for example, when perceiving that a person tumbles downstairs and remains motionless at the end of the fall, might be impressed by several different communicative aspects of this incident. Referring to the physical sphere, the conclusion may be warranted that the person was injured. With reference to the intrapersonal system of the victim, the inference is made that certain processes within the mind of the accident-bearer may have been altered or arrested, and that the person has lost consciousness. Pertinent to the interpersonal relation, the conclusion is warranted that the person needs help; and in social terms, though not immediately, certain repercussions can be expected which might deal with lawsuits, establishment of rules for accident prevention, and the like. Thus any change in the state of an organism can be viewed from varied standpoints and can be registered consciously or unconsciously.

If actions of human beings and animals have communicative

aspects, so also do plants and objects convey a message to the person who perceives them. It takes but the fraction of a second for our organism to perceive a multitude of stimuli, and most scientific descriptions of perceptive phenomena run into insurmountable difficulties when an attempt is made to describe the processes involved. A brief illustration may serve as an example. When our attention is attracted by the sight of a red rose, we conceive its splendor under the influence of messages transmitted to us through several channels. First we see, then we smell, and eventually after approaching the rose, we can touch the flower. The scientific description of these three steps would run into many hundreds of pages. Starting with the assessment of the color, the wave length of the reflected light, for example, could be specified as being around 7,000 Angstrom units. Thereafter the tint or shade of the color, the angle of reflection, the position and nature of the original source of light, its brightness, the surface texture and the color of the contrasting background, and many other features would have to be studied to complete the scientific description of the processes related to light alone. Botanical specifications of the family and species of the rose bush, identification of the time and duration of the process of blooming, would embrace some of the plant biological aspects of the investigation. Specifications of the odor emitted by the blossom, the number and type of insects attracted, and their effectiveness in seed dispersion might follow next. Chemical analysis of the constituent parts of the rose tissues or an assessment of the soil or weather conditions might head other chapters of the scientific study. Finally, after exhausting consideration of the rose, and of the conditions under which it bloomed, the investigation would finally reach the human being who perceives the rose. Name, age, sex, and other specifications would be needed to identify us, the individual observer. Study of our physical health and assessment of our visual apparatus would probably precede the psychological investigation of our past experiences, in particular those with flowers and roses. Psychological probing might reveal traces of previous events which enabled us to focus upon the rose rather than upon the structure of the wall in the background or upon a dog playing near by. Further elaboration might reveal the purposes that we might have had in focusing upon roses, either as decoration of the buttonhole in the lapel, as an arrangement on our desk, or maybe as a present for a beloved one. And after all this long and tedious scientific preparation and accumulation of information regarding the rose and the human being who perceived it, we would have to be concerned with that split second which it took to see the rose, and those few seconds more which were necessary to walk towards it.

The reader will readily understand that no scientist is able to describe all the things that might have acted as stimuli or all the possible reactions that a person might have had in that situation. Nevertheless, a neutral observer, sitting on a bench near by, and observing the act of approach and of picking the rose, might infer a number of things from his own experiences in similar situations. He might conclude that we possess a readiness—or shall we say a preference—for that particular rose at that particular time in that particular situation. Let us say that the act of picking the rose had for us the significance of satisfying a desire and of providing us with a present, while for the observer it constituted an expressive act which transmitted to him information about ourself and the rose as well as about the total situation which was conducive to this act. To him, the observer, the only thing that was obvious was the combination of a particular stimulus, the rose, with a particular kind of response, the picking. This combination of a particular stimulus with a particular response we have called a value. For the observer, the choice of this act indicated to him that at that particular moment no other act could take place, though, for example, we might have walked by, heading for the dog without even noticing the rose. For ourselves who proceeded to pick the rose, the act created a precedent which might influence future actions and which in itself was a sequel to previous experiences of ours. Regardless of whether we were aware of our choice, and regardless of whether we knew the motivating reasons for our actions, we, as well as any observer, would agree that at the instant we picked the rose we conveyed a message to others. And this message certainly carried the meaning that within the context of this situation we valued—above all—a rose.

For purposes of communication, then, any action constitutes a message to ourselves as well as to others. Within the framework of communication, the expression and transmission of values—that is, actions denoting a choice—occupy a central place. A value conveys not only information about the choice made, but also relays information about the things that could have been chosen but were not selected. The ability to select, to maximize or minimize certain aspects of perception, are features which characterize our communication center. Furthermore, this center possesses the faculty of retaining traces of past experiences. Obviously not the action itself, but a symbolic representation, is retained, which has the function of representing within the human organism a small-scale model of all the events which have been experienced in the past.

Creation of new things and adaptation through molding of the surroundings distinguishes man from all other creatures. This gift, which the organicist calls "brain" and which the mentalist refers to as "psyche," is localized nowhere. With no anatomical structure of its own, none the less it needs for its functioning the sum total of all the cells and properties of the organism. To integrate parts into a whole, to magnify, minimize, or discard events, to evaluate the past and to anticipate the future, to create that which never before existed, such are the functions of the center. The infant, when born, is vested with all these potentialities; their exploitation, however, depends upon experiences and circumstances. Equipped with an insatiable desire for a search for the new, the exploration of things and people grinds permanent and indelible grooves into the center of the child. Imprints become experiences when events are registered, and traces remain available for future reference. Little by little, information is acquired through representation of outside events in the mind of the child. Happenings in and around a person are recorded in codified form, and complementation of immediate impressions with traces of the past facilitates a selective response. The individual is said to have learned when discriminating reactions as well as anticipation of events indicate mastery of self and surroundings.

The expansion of the maturing individual is controlled by

biological limitations which in turn delineate the extension in space of the system of communication. Man's genetic endowment forces him to seek social relations, while his early development and his first social contacts will in part determine the way he is going to use (145) and eventually refine his means of communication. Man is born of a mother. After his birth, certain death would embrace the infant unless it were fed, clothed, and sheltered. The severance of the umbilical cord is but the first step towards achieving independence. The infant's struggle to acquire an identity of his own requires some fifteen or twenty years. During this time, the growing child, at first helpless and immobilized, little by little learns to explore the world and to undertake ventures on his own. Tedious codification of events leading to the accumulation of a vast mass of information and acquisition of the "know-how" pertaining to the use of this information enables the child to relinquish gradually the help received from parents and protectors. When biological maturation and social learning have progressed sufficiently, the child is equipped to set out on his own and to continue the battle for life with a reasonable chance of survival. Now even more than before, communication with fellow men becomes a necessity, since information about the self, others, and the surroundings has to be kept up to date. The state of maturity has been reached when finally communication and cooperation with contemporaries has replaced the former reliance upon physical and emotional assistance from elders.

Man's concept of the world is acquired through social interaction (114) and communication, and these acquired views are the foundations upon which will rest the future organization of his surroundings. The shaping of things in the environment distinguishes man from all other living creatures. Man has mastered his physical limitations by extension in space and time. His voice, audible within a few hundred yards at best, now can encompass the globe and perhaps beyond. His movements in space, under primitive conditions, perhaps extended a few hundred miles; now they embrace the whole world and possibly more. The creation of script, the construction of man-made shelters, and the use of design enables messages from times past to reach future generations. The invention of time-binding mass communication led to the formation of a cumulative body of knowledge. Information accumulated in the course of centuries became the ground upon which were erected new object systems and events which eventually developed an existence of their own. In contrast to the animal, the human being has to face not only other people but messages and productions of the past as well. The inventions of man, frequently designed in the name of progress and survival, may undermine his biological foundations. Whether in the end the creations of man will improve his lot or result in his own modification or in his total annihilation remains to be seen. Be that as it may, at the root of all man-made events stands his ability to communicate, which is the foundation upon which cooperation is built.

Cooperation is closely linked to those characteristics which make man a gregarious creature. Thus man does not live alone. Usually he is surrounded by parents, mate, and offspring, and he seeks the company of contemporaries. In the fold of the family, the clan, the group, or, in the widest sense of the word, the herd, he feels secure. Here, the threatening experiences can be shared, and through pooling of information and cooperation of forces he can master adverse events. Reliance upon other members of the group increases his chances for survival in a troubled world. The first experience of being helped and raised by the mother or other members of the group induces man to trust or fear people. If trust and confidence prevail, he will seek the help of others; if fear predominates he will dominate or avoid others. But regardless of the motive, be it for the sake of sharing, avoiding, conquering, or destroying, he always needs other people.

Man has to move. As the infant acquires mastery of space, locomotion is soon supplemented by other means of transportation. In boats, on the backs of animals, on wheels, or on wings, the exploration of the world is carried on. Movement in space facilitates the acquisition and dissemination of information and the satisfaction of needs. Transportation and communication are thus so intimately linked that distinction is hardly possible.

In his exploration of space, in his quest for mastery, and in his need for food, shelter, and a mate, man will meet dangers and perhaps interference from others. Man and animal alike are alarmed at the sight of danger, and anything is threatening which, by their experience, is not known to be harmless. In animals, alarm—that is, impending readiness for events to come—is told in many ways: the lion tosses his mane and roars, the fiddler crab brandishes a bright red claw, while the moor hen utters a harsh "krek." A cat when chased by a dog seeks refuge in a tree, its fur erect, claws thrust into the bark, hissing at the growling canine below. The cat's body spells readiness for any future action if a change in the situation should occur; when prowling and stalking a mouse, it will patiently wait for hours for the opportune jump which will spell doom to the outwitted rodent.

While the alarmed animal has the choice of fight, flight, or playing possum, the human being has one additional opportunity. Constructive action, designed to eliminate the source of danger, long-term planning with the intent of preventing a recurrence of the danger, and pooling of information with subsequent cooperation with other humans are the unique privileges of man. Communication for the purpose of sharing and transmission of information to obtain the views of others provides help for the alarmed person. When fight, flight, playing possum, and communication are barred, the readiness of the body for action cannot be consummated. The continuous alarm becomes a permanent state, which is referred to as anxiety. Eventually the overtaxation of mind and body will gradually lead to a breakdown of integrated functioning. The individual is then psychologically and physically sick; the focusing of protracted attention upon the impending danger monopolizes the mental resources, and perpetual readiness of the body results in anxiety and fatigue. Unawareness of other circumstances which might require immediate attention and the inability to mobilize the worn-out body for maximal effort eventually defeat the individual in situations which otherwise he could easily have mastered. Even then, communication is a helpful procedure. The process of talking, though not an act of great physical expenditure for the individual, will absorb the overflow of readiness, and eventually a person is again enabled to find his bearings. This interpersonal process constitutes the core of any type of psychotherapy.

The human being's need for social action is the moving force which compels him to master the tools of communication. Without these his ability to gather information is imperiled and gratification of vital needs is threatened. The superiority of a person within his group is determined in the first instance by skillful use of his means of communication; to receive information and to give that which others need, to possess a workable concept of events, and to act accordingly, marks the successful man.

THE MORE COMPLEX SYSTEMS OF COMMUNICATION

The simpler systems of communication are characterized by the fact that participants can trace a message from its origin to its destination; therefore it is possible, though not necessary, for the participants to recognize and correct distortions. In such a system the circular characteristics become obvious, transmission of messages and effect achieved are closely connected in space and time, and the participants get the feeling that they are able to master the situation. The simpler systems are, by and large, symmetrical systems; all participating persons are equipped with receivers, transmitters, and communication centers which enable them to retain and to evaluate information. At birth, the infant enters an asymmetrical system of communication, because his own communication machinery is as yet not fully developed; however, a healthy human environment will bring about a gradual rectification of this asymmetry, and as soon as the biological maturity of the child will permit, symmetrical communication will be initiated. We shall later elaborate upon the fact that if children are raised in a human environment in which symmetrical systems of communication prevail, they are likely to be mentally healthy, and that if unfortunate circumstances force a person to remain in asymmetrical systems, disturbances of communication will occur.

The larger and more complex systems of communication which include a group of people or several groups are usually asymmetrical. The flow of messages either emerges from a center or converges to a center; in such systems either many persons communicate with one person, or one person communicates with many. If, for example, a politician addresses the nation, he proceeds with one-way communication in which his listeners have no opportunity for an immediate reply. Likewise when a governmental agency submits its field reports to the head of the department, the executive is unable to give individual replies to the queries of his informants or constituents. The physical limitations of a human being's receiving system are such that only a limited number of messages can be taken care of within one day. If the number of incoming messages exceeds the capacity of the receiver, each message must be abstracted, and the abstractions grouped until the receiver can master the number of entities to be considered. From the abstract conclusions the executive is frequently unable to evaluate the original messages correctly; and since he is rarely in a position to talk personally to the senders of the original messages, he is acting primarily as a receiver in a one-way communication system. These asymmetrical systems, which we have termed "group networks," are characterized by the fact that either the source or the destination of the messages is anonymous, and that correction of the messages is therefore delayed. In order to compensate for the asymmetries of such systems, efficient executives have developed short-circuit methods to avoid the progressive steps of abstraction, and therefore distortion of meaning, on the one hand, and the echelon of command which adds to or subtracts from the original message, on the other hand. Thus a commanding general will appear at the front to get first-hand information, personally, and the emissaries of foreign governments frequently report in person in order to avoid the distortions which occur when information passes through various hands.

The most complex communication network is encountered when we consider a cultural network in which many persons communicate with many others. Here both the origin and the destination of the messages remain anonymous, and therefore correction of messages becomes impossible. As a result of this situation, the individual feels helpless to cope with the messages with which he is swamped. He searches in vain for the source of origin or destination of the messages. Knowledge of these fixed points in a communication network would, through feedback, enable participants to modify their own messages and correctly interpret the messages of others. In recent times, for example, most citizens have been eagerly ready to do something in order to avoid war, but from time to time they have been unable to escape the feeling that war was inevitable. The helplessness experienced by people when they are swamped with rumors and anonymous messages is probably due to the fact that every person has a need for personal acknowledgment of his or her message. Therefore one might state that insecurity is the direct result of anonymity of origin or destination of messages, with the implication that the individual feels paralyzed if correction of erroneous interpretations is impossible.

THE CULTURAL NETWORK

An individual who is unaware of the existence of larger cultural systems will accept events as natural. If, however, a person is aware of historical and cultural events, he is frustrated by the fact that he is unable to fully understand the processes that take place. Let us therefore attempt to shed some light upon this matter. It is the anthropologist's task to study such superpersonal systems; the statements which he tends to make about a "culture" consist primarily of generalizations about people and groups of people. What people do and say and what they have done and said comprise the bulk of his data. "Culture" as such cannot be observed directly; it only exists in the form of generalized statements made by social scientists about people, which include not only the specific organizational patterns of people in groups, but also their judicial and economic problems, their language and systems of symbolization, their conventions and traditions, and all objects, buildings, and monuments which convey some message from the past (147).

To the native of a primitive tribe who has spent his whole life in the same place, it seems quite natural that things are as they are. However, the anthropologist recognizes, from his knowledge of other places and people, that some of the observed features are unique. Because he is a stranger he is able to see what the native takes for granted. However, accustomed to seeing and doing things in a manner different from that of the native, the anthropologist meets at each step a new problem. His lack of familiarity with this particular culture is revealed when he wishes to communicate with the natives, when he involuntarily violates some basic rule, or when he just wishes to order a meal. Likewise in the process of discovering a new "culture," all travelers are forced to deduce some principles by which they can understand the natives. This is the exact position which confronts the American cultural anthropologist when he wishes to learn something about Bali, or the English anthropologist when he studies America. And the same position confronts the social scientist when he explores a group of people other than his own. Evidently the process of making generalizations about the behavior of people is necessary when a stranger finds himself surrounded by people who differ from him in many respects. It does not matter whether he is a traveler in a foreign country or a lawyer among physicians; the principle remains the same.

In general, the members of a given culture or subculture are remarkably unaware of the premises which they observe in their system of communication. Nobody is really able to evaluate his own utterances in terms of the greater system of which he is a part. Though some people may act in perfect accordance with their respective cultural principles, and some of the natives may even state premises with great explicitness, the formulation of the premises which are the basis of a cultural network can only be undertaken by a stranger or by a native who has lived in cultural systems other than his own. Only by the experience of contrast can the observer acquire the necessary awareness and perspective to make relevant generalizations; these generalizations constitute a dictionary which enables the person to translate the signals received into the system of codification with which he is familiar.

We mentioned above the helplessness which people experience when they cannot trace the origin and destination of a message. This implies, however, that people are aware of the fact that messages can be traced to human sources. In each culture there exist beliefs and traditions which cannot be traced to human sources. These messages are accepted by the population as if they were messages from God, or messages from a mythological figure, or as if they were an expression of the nature of things. But regardless of the supposed source to which these messages are attributed, the outstanding feature is that there is no recourse, no reply, and no possibility of correction on the part of the native. The anthropologist, in contrast, is aware that in another culture, perhaps, this particular area of belief is modifiable, while other areas may be inaccessible to correction. The areas which are inaccessible to correction we shall call cultural mass communication.

Thus one can say that cultural mass communication influences every citizen living within its reach. Examples of such mass communication are found in the messages which governments and leaders direct toward the people. Here, one or more persons send messages to the people at large which may be in the form of proclamations, broadcasts, plays, films, newspapers, articles, and the like. A characteristic feature of these communications is the multiple and often indefinite character of the emitting agency. The communications usually originate in an institution or administrative department, and by the time a speech or a play has been made public it has been worked upon by many persons. It is no longer a message from one individual to another, but is a message from many to many, and in the end so many people have participated that the process must be labeled a true "mass communication." Children are continually exposed to such mass communications in terms of the radio, television, the comics, and, last but not least, the climate of opinion of the family itself.

A second kind of event to be considered under the heading of cultural communication is the transmission of statements about tradition and statements about the conventional procedures pertaining to ceremonies, trade customs, health, child-raising practices, and the like. In contrast to the *ad hoc* character of the messages discussed above, information pertaining to custom constitutes in most societies a more constant, though slowly changing reiteration of the mass communications of the past. The spectator can observe how information whose origin is frequently anonymous is handed down from generation to generation and can note its effects on the behavior of people living in the present era.

A third type of event to be included under the title of cultural communication is found in the material, man-made objects and arrangements of objects with which people surround themselves. Because of the dimensions and duration of construction, cathedrals, dams, roads, and dwellings are beyond the scope of any one individual. Once again, these object systems become mass communications in which both originators and recipients of the messages frequently remain anonymous.

A fourth type of event of societal dimensions is found in the system of symbolization and language which a person must learn if he wishes to participate within a given group. Not only the systems of symbolization but also the subtle shadings in the meanings of symbols have to be mastered. Every citizen learns through the impact of mass communication how to interpret the meaning of messages not only by assessing the content, but above all by watching certain cues related to the manner of presentation. Punctuation, emphasis, attention-getting, assignment of roles, and the expression of emotion can all be seen as messages about communication, which guide the recipient in his understanding—his decodification and evaluation of the messages. The meaning of the word "please," for example, or the significance of the voice raised in a certain context, are part of the shared culture, learned from the outer social matrix, either from mass communication or from personal experience in dealing with other persons of the same culture. The rules for communication about communication—which are also the rules defining human relationship—are presumed to be common to many people, whereas the simpler primary content of the message is presumed to be a matter of the immediate moment and special to the speaker.

Now, it goes without saying that what is presumed to be personal and ephemeral is more subject to change than the more basic patterns, which are presumed to be either absolute or at least shared by large numbers of persons. The individual's freedom of action and self-correction is presumed to be relatively great at a personal level. He sees the effects of his actions, he can correct them, and he can relate cause and effect. But difficulties arise in regard to those ideas which the individual assumes to be shared by large numbers of people. The person in question may be exceedingly deviant from other people in his communicative habits, and may have his own special rules for interpreting communicative overtones. Yet he unconsciously assumes that these rules are shared, and that they are a part of the inevitable and unchanging nature of life. Such an individual is the psychiatric patient. The difficult task of therapy at this level is to lead the patient to the discovery that his inarticulate and usually unconscious assumptions about human relationships, about communication, and about the culture in which he lives are incorrect, and to help him learn that mass communications are man-made and that they can be changed.

These unconscious assumptions about the universality of rules of communication are made not only by individuals, but by groups of people and nations as a whole. In this context, the outbreak of a war can be viewed as that moment in which people realize their isolation in terms of communication. In resorting to armed intervention they force the opponent to do the same, namely to resort to war. This procedure eliminates their isolation inasmuch as both nations then follow a common system, that of violence and war. This has in itself an equalizing effect upon the systems of communication of both nations, inasmuch as they now share a system of communication common to both. After a varying period of time and with the leveling effect of war, they then are able to live again without war, assuming that the opponent, having gone through all the same hardships, now shares with them the same rules of communication.

A considerable amount of literature has been compiled by anthropologists, psychologists, and sociologists about the impact of such mass communications upon the individual. Essentially these mass communications can be considered to form a social matrix in which human relations take place. The manner in which this matrix influences individual and interpersonal behavior can be understood best by introducing the concept of value premise.

VALUE PREMISE AND COMMUNICATION

The term "value" is rather commonly used in popular speech and is closely linked with two notions: that value can be ascribed to any object or action, and that value is a quantity which makes possible comparative evaluation. Any object or action can supposedly be compared with any other object or action, when values are substituted for the idea of either. In terms of these notions, value is a device which renders incomparable things commensurable; for example, people link price with almost every sort of action and commodity; thus, five dollars' worth of baby shoes can be rated against five dollars' worth of whiskey. Value is also a device by which closely similar things can be differentiated; one brand of whiskey can be preferred to another because its price is a few cents more or a few cents less. For the purposes of our study, however, the word "value" will be used with a more general and less quantitative meaning (124).

This wider meaning of the concept of value can be derived from the somewhat simpler notion of preference. "Preference" always refers to an organism's reaction to two or more possibilities which have been perceived. These possibilities refer on the one hand to a series of perceived stimuli and on the other hand to a series of anticipated reactions of the organism. In order to facilitate a decision in the face of these multiple choices, the organism subdivides the perceived stimuli and the anticipated reactions into groups. Through a series of complicated processes, the individual finally comes out with a statement of preference. Such a statement of preference we shall term a value.

Through statements of preference, the inner workings of the mind of a person are revealed. Frequently only two choices are present as alternatives. Thus "death" and "dishonor" may be linked as alternatives, or "whiskey" and "baby shoes," or "baseball" and "softball." In these instances the choice situation is clear; but most of the time the choices are so numerous that they cannot be arranged as simple alternatives. It seems that in the life of an individual, his own actions, the external objects with which he is surrounded, the events in which he participates, and even those in which he is a spectator—all these are arranged in a network of preferences.

These ramifying systems or networks of preference that concern us in the present study are the core of all processes of communication. For example, if we as person B hear person A make a verbal statement or see a gesture of his or simply watch this person proceeding in his activities, the following implications occur to us, aided by our assumptions regarding the speaker and our knowledge of his culture:

First that within the social field in which A operates a large number of possible stimuli have arisen; second, that A, operating in this field, has perceived a segment of these stimuli but that it is impossible to specify the perceived stimuli; third, that A possesses a number of ways in which to respond; fourth, that the response which A finally makes is the end product of a complicated process. Neither A nor we as B are sure which stimuli have been perceived nor what range of responses has been considered. Finally, all we see is a preferential action on the part of A. This action implies the notion that a stimulus, out of a large field of stimuli, was linked with a response out of a field of responses. Thus it is well to remember that in daily communication any preferential or value statement is not only a message of that which was chosen, but implicitly evokes in the listener certain associations referring to what might have been perceived, the courses which might have been chosen, and judgments about what ought to have been done. As a matter of fact, this implied background is the feature which gives meaning to any statement, and both speaker and listener make liberal use of it; "you know what I mean" is an expression which illustrates this phenomenon, invoking either the common cultural background or the listener's previous experience of the speaker's system of values.

Several assumptions regarding the other person's psychological processes are made when people converse with each other. We, as B, for example, assume that when A has perceived the various alternatives, he will compare one alternative with another; in other words, we assume that A will arrive at some action or statement in which preference is present—either overt or implicit. Furthermore, we attribute to A the ability to rate hetero-geneous elements—at least in pairs—on a homogeneous scale. "Comparison" implies that however different the items, some common denominator can be found. This inferred psychological process includes not only our considerations pertaining to the nature of the stimuli and A's possible responses but also includes the idea that A has had certain past experiences. In daily lan-guage, the term "justification" denotes certain personal deliber-ations which serve the purpose of matching present events with past experiences. In this manner contemplated action is matched with ideas which refer to commonly accepted practices. The as-sumptions we make about A therefore refer to intrapersonal processes, among which we include perception, comparison, justification, and evaluation, which are assumed to lead either to an overt statement of preference or to an action from which we, as observer, can deduce preference.

At this point it seems necessary to recapitulate what we have said about the function of the culture in interpersonal relations. We state simply that a value premise is a generalization made by an observer about another person's perceptions and actions. The observer imputes or "projects" these generalizations upon the other person. Conversely, the person who engages in some action —be it speech, gesture, or other movement—does so in order to become accessible to the observer. In doing so, a person expresses his preference system. A actually causes B to draw in-ferences about his, A's, intrapersonal process which would other-wise be inaccessible. The observer is encouraged to fill in the other's meaning from his own reservoir of information. It is only by means of this filling-in that the observer is able to un-derstand the message. These "fill-ins" are, of course, derived from cultural mass communications to which an individual has been exposed. Persons who have been raised within the same cultural system speak more or less the same language and possess more or less the same values. They may differ or even argue about preferences, but they do understand each other and by and large they will agree as to which items can appropriately be compared, and they are alike in their concepts regarding the "common denominator" mentioned above.

Understanding (169) consists largely of perceiving a person's action and deducing from it the series of intrapersonal processes of which it is the end result. It is quite evident that the more correct the inferences, the more the two people will come to possess common information. Knowledge about the other person can be acquired in several ways; the first way consists of living with an individual over a long period of time. Through continued accumulation of information on the one hand and through repeated exposure to similar events on the other, the two people learn to draw correct inferences about each other's behavior. However, this method is time-consuming and often not practical, because in daily life we have to confer with a great many people whom we have never seen before. In spite of not knowing intimately the majority of the people whom we encounter, we possess some *a priori* information about their system of values if we have information about the culture in which they have lived. If these other persons are members of our own culture, this information will be rather detailed.

In Chapters 4, 5, and 6 we shall dwell in greater detail upon this *a priori* information which people share who dwell in the American sector of the orbit of Western civilization. The value premises which govern communication in America—the social matrix—will be presented by assuming that an English-speaking traveler explores America for the first time in his life, and is amazed by the many things he does not understand (32), (47), (65), (86), (95), (102), (157), (167). Some of these observations are common knowledge among foreigners, but the native is frequently unable to verbalize these very same aspects. The American native implicitly understands and acts upon all these cues and never has to give them a second thought (7), (9), (49), (69), (82), (112), (175). But as soon as the American-born psychiatrist deals with therapy and rehabilitation—that is, when he tries to improve the means of communication of the patient— he must become more consciously aware of the nature of the communication which prevails between him and the patient. While in daily life people continually communicate on the basis of very incomplete information, this procedure is rather unsatisfactory when a psychiatrist is attempting to carry out therapy.

Incomplete information may suffice in daily life because immediately following action will fill in some of the missing information. However, in therapy, where attempts are made to change the system of communication itself, more complete information has to be available for a successful conclusion of the task. Therefore, before we proceed to discuss the nature of the information inherent in the social matrix, we shall review in the next chapter how psychiatrists have to rely upon information bearing upon values and communication in order to help their patients.

3 · COMMUNICATION AND MENTAL ILLNESS: A Psychiatric Approach

By Jurgen Ruesch

PEOPLE LIVE, but successful living is an art which is not mastered by all. Those who feel this failure—the patients—seek improvement, and those who believe that they know about failure—the therapists—attempt to induce improvement. A give-and-take develops when patients and therapists meet, and the events which occur under such circumstances are referred to as psychotherapy. But therapeutic happenings are met in all walks of life. In social relations it does not matter who is in need of help and who provides the assistance. It is not necessary, and sometimes not even wise, that people know they are being helped. What counts is the feeling of diminishing failure in the one who suffers and the knowledge of this change in the one who helps. The feeling of relief experienced after successful communication molds people in such a way that they begin to seek the companionship of others. At one time the participants may be mother and child, at another, doctor and patient; in one instance it may be teacher and pupil, and in another, worshiper and spiritual adviser. Each of these teams is likely to have a different set of words and symbols and their own scientific or philosophical systems to describe what has happened; however, the nature of the events remains similar, being always an experience which occurs in relation with other people. It is the task of psychiatry to help those who have failed to experience successful communication, and it is the aim of psychiatry as a scientific discipline to gain information about the nature of these failures and to formulate remedial measures.

A psychotherapist approaches human behavior with the clear understanding that he is not only interested in studying and observing people's actions but also that he is specifically concentrating upon those aspects of behavior which in the course of therapy are likely to change. The therapist uses his knowledge of human behavior for the purposes of improving the health of the patient. Whatever his training and his specific beliefs may be, as a therapist he seeks to influence the behavior of those who come to him for assistance. In contrast to the natural scientist, who investigates nature and concentrates upon that which is, the therapist is interested essentially in that which is going to be; potentialities of development rather than fixation of the *status quo* are visualized as the aim of therapeutic endeavors. However, this point of view is not universally shared by all; there are still many psychiatrists who view deviant behavior and mental disease as a *curiosum* which has to be catalogued and housed, displaying an attitude which is very similar to that of the naturalist. In addition to these two types of specialists, we have to mention also those psychiatrists whose primary interest lies in the fields of administration, social or physiological research or court work, and who occupy positions which can be likened neither to that of the therapist nor to that of the naturalist. A brief sketch of the psychiatric scene will illustrate these divergent points of view.

THE CONTEMPORARY PSYCHIATRIC SCENE

Perhaps the most important influence upon psychotherapeutic thinking was exerted by Freud. This fact is documented by the number of followers who, in their adherence to the orthodox psychoanalytic system, constitute a living monument to his genius (54). In addition, other influences have shaped considerably the thinking of American therapists. We have to mention Adler, Jung, Rank, Reich and Stekel (122), who at one time or another were associated with the Freudian movement and who all have their followers in this country. Besides these Austrian, Swiss, and German influences, there have also been repercussions from the writings of Charcot, Janet, and Bernheim of France (83), (84). We may group together the various European psycho- therapeutic schools as constituting one root in the present com- plex picture of American psychiatry and note that a second root is found in a school which originated in this country. It antedated some of the therapeutic movements in Europe and is associated with the name of Adolph Meyer (101). Meyer, though himself a European of Swiss origin, attempted to integrate the more structural thinking of the Europeans with American notions of process and change. He was the first to state the importance of behavioral reactions and to stress the concept of adjustment to life situations, thus introducing fluidity into the rather static notions of psychiatry of his time. A third root of modern Ameri- can psychiatry derives from academic psychology, reflecting the various trends of psychological thinking (44). Names such as Watson, Prince, James, McDougall, are familiar to all (121), while in more recent times those schools which emphasize gestalt psychology (89), and more recent experimental work on condi- tioning (100), (128) and learning (75), (119), have had a con- siderable influence. A fourth root (125) of American psychiatry can be found in the state hospital system as it developed in the course of the nineteenth century (186), while a fifth root is to be found in clinical medicine, physiology, and neuropathology (39), (40), (58).

Today, then, the value premises which govern American psy- chotherapy can be traced to their five historical roots: psycho- analysis, psychobiology, experimental as well as social psychology, state hospital psychiatry, and medicine. A synthesis of the various components resulted in premises which indicate that European concepts are being adapted to the American scene and social science concepts are being mixed with purely physiological ap- proaches. Among the modern American trends of thought one would have to mention psychosomatic medicine (137), (141), (150). The efforts of Dunbar (50), (51), Alexander and French (4), Weiss and English (174), and others constitute an attempt at integrating psychoanalytic concepts with physiological findings met with in the practice of clinical medicine (2). Another attempt to adapt psychoanalysis to the present needs of psychiatry was made by Alexander and French (3) in their *Psychoanalytic Therapy,* in which they advocated fewer interviews, avoidance of intense transference reactions, and other short cuts. Similarly Rogers (133) proposed a method entitled "non-directive counseling," which is directed toward a discussion of current adjustment problems as selected by the "client." An attempt at correcting the traditional isolation of psychiatry from the other social sciences was made by Sullivan (160), Horney (76), Fromm (56), Kardiner (85), Ruesch (140), (143), and others, calling attention to the social matrix in which both patient and psychiatrist operate. The Washington school of psychiatry (120), for example, is built upon Sullivan's premise that interpersonal relations rather than the intrapsychic structure of the patient ought to be the principle concern of the modern psychiatrist. Among other important trends, child psychology, child development, and child guidance must be mentioned (6), (71). They developed as the result of a synthesis of two principal trends —Freud's emphasis upon childhood events on the one hand, and the American emphasis upon family life on the other. Theories and observations pertaining to childhood events fell in America upon fertile ground because the life of the American family is especially organized around the child and anything that benefits children will be readily absorbed by the public.

Considering the operational aspects of American therapy, one must state that the expressive type of therapy is preferred to the suppressive (57). The latter would obviously conflict with the American ideology of equality, in which freeing the individual from any identifiable oppressive authority is a foremost goal. Therapies (5) related to expression other than verbal are found in such procedures as occupational therapy (70), play therapy (46), psychodrama (115), (116), music therapy (99), and finger painting (156). The premises related to social manipulation in the American culture are expressed in psychiatric social work (55) and other attempts at environmental manipulation. The cultural premises of engineering and emphasis upon bodily health can be recognized in those methods which directly manipulate and influence the body, such as progressive relaxation (81), dieting (154), and the like. Group therapy (68) is obviously an expression of the American premise of sociability and the value set upon getting along in a group. Narcosynthesis (77) emerged from an attempt to combine hypnotism (30), (183) with drug action; this method was thought to save time and effort and was widely applied in emergency situations during World War II (66), (67).

The combined efforts of the various therapeutic schools, teaching institutions, and other bodies interested in therapy and the prevention of mental disease have brought about some change in public opinion about psychiatry. Today these diversified influences have united their forces and are organized and subsumed under the heading of mental health. Due to this widespread mental health movement we witness in America an integrative process in which psychoanalysis, psychobiology, state hospital procedures, and medicine are welded more and more into a unit (118), (129). Growing cooperation (104) between psychiatrists, psychologists, anthropologists, social workers, public health officers, welfare workers, judges, and police officers, as well as medical practitioners, demonstrates the diffusion of the concepts underlying mental health. Community, state, and federal legislative and executive bodies become increasingly aware of the growing need for steps which will take care of problems of maladjustment; then bodies of responsible men progressively appropriate more money for mental hospitals, teaching, and research. More and more scientific study and therapeutic effort are directed at the rehabilitation of criminals, juvenile delinquents, the blind and the deaf, the accident-prone, spastic children, and those suffering from infantile paralysis (12). Industry is tackling its own problems, and in no other country in the world is industrial psychiatry so advanced as in America (132). Last but not least, racial prejudice, slum clearance, and even intolerance between religious groups have become the concern of those interested in mental health. The cooperative effect of various groups has resulted in a progressive breakdown of the rigid separation of scientific and therapeutic disciplines. Through a general process of elbow rubbing, responsible persons expose themselves to different views, and such diffusion of information has a direct impact upon the fate of the deviant person. Whether it is in terms of cultural, physical, or psychological care, more and more chronic invalids and underprivileged people are today rehabilitated by the newly founded health divisions of community, government, and scientific institutions.

The effect of the American culture, with its premise of equality and its emphasis on health, is to diffuse knowledge and obliterate individual differences. At the same time it promotes the formation of pressure groups which compete for supremacy and power. Psychiatry is not exempt from these tendencies. While in Europe this competition is expressed in terms of divergent ideological views which either are not organized at all or become the supreme credo of some totalitarian regime, in America ideologies are advanced as a moral screen for the attainment of power. The latter procedure warrants, of course, efficient political organization in terms of societies, associations, or groups which exert pressure and share among the members the spoils which have been gained.

Any association or organization will more or less conform to the models of organization which are provided by the political system of a given country. This statement is not meant to be taken literally, inasmuch as these similarities become pronounced only on a rather abstract level. However, if the reader will keep in mind the description of the system of checks and balances (see p. 153) he will understand the similarity to which we refer. No idea, whether it derives from religious, social, or individual thinking, can escape political exploitation if it becomes known at all. There will always be somebody who will utilize such an idea in the furtherance of his quest for power. Napoleon attempted to conquer the world in the name of the French Revolution, and the Crusades were conducted in the name of Christianity. And all too frequently, those eager followers of a productive idea have to resort to methods which destroy the very notion which they attempt to introduce.

At first an idea is usually the property of a single individual; later it may spread but is still distinctly segregated from the rest of the popular body of knowledge, until finally it becomes the center of political organization. As the years go by it becomes institutionalized, and only when the official organization which surrounds the ideas has been corrupted and disintegrates, does the idea, perhaps in a modified form, become public property. The time lag between the introduction of an idea and its acceptance by the public at large has been calculated to amount to more than two hundred years (186).

In psychiatry, the collection of a cumulative body of knowledge to which a large number of anonymous scientists contribute is just beginning. At present we are really still in the second stage of development, with its emphasis upon individual schools and segregation. Each prominent member of the psychiatric profession who has either invented a theory or introduced a special kind of therapeutic practice tends to found a new school of thought. Today we still find psychiatric schools tied up with the names of individuals, bitterly fighting rival schools, tied up with the names of other individuals. The differences mentioned are usually related to divergent views and theories rather than to divergent operations; as a matter of fact, one might even go so far as to say that there exists considerably more agreement as far as therapeutic operations are concerned than is apparent from the theoretical discussions. It appears as if psychiatrists progressively tend to agree on operational definitions, becoming more tolerant of each other's viewpoints and behaving more like engineers than like artists.

The importance attributed to change by the American people, the existing emphasis upon engineering and applied science, the optimism of the American people with regard to social improvement, are the foundations upon which psychotherapy could develop. At present, the diversified schools have incorporated some of these values in their respective schemes and are in the process of changing their theoretical formulations. These formulations originated in various places in Europe and had their roots in a variety of historical and social events. America is not only the melting pot of nations but is also the place where compromises are made with regard to theoretical formulations; theories for theory's sake are abandoned, idiosyncrasies are renounced, special positions and viewpoints are modified, and formulations are offered for the purpose of practical application.

THE PRESENT STATE OF PSYCHIATRIC THEORY

This brief sketch of the contemporary psychiatric scene might suffice to illustrate the present state of organization of the field of psychiatry. Now we shall turn our attention to psychiatric theory. To discuss the various theoretical systems which are used to explain deviant behavior is beyond the scope of this volume; and furthermore, it would only repeat that which is well known. Instead we shall call attention to the fact that a grave schism exists between psychiatric theory and psychiatric practice, to the extent that frequently theory and practice seem to be rather loosely connected, if not contradictory. In order to illustrate this peculiar paradox an attempt will be made to reduce the multifarious psychiatric theories to a few basic premises. We shall argue that these premises cannot be combined into a satisfactory psychiatric system because they derive from various historical periods, each with a different focus and purpose; therefore existing psychiatric theories are unsatisfactory when used to explain modern therapeutic techniques. We shall argue further that, inasmuch as modern therapies are concerned with expression and the improvement of the means of communication of the patient, the theory of communication is best fitted to explain therapeutic procedures.

Lineal and circular systems. In the extreme mechanistic emphasis of the eighteenth and nineteenth centuries (147) the causal chains for which scientists searched were, almost without exception, lineal, branching, or converging. The question "why," the belief in single causation (29), and the stress upon the problems of etiology and assessment of disease overdetermined the answers which were obtained. A chain of events spaced in time or a set of conditions patterned in space were linked together to build a theory of causality, and what preceded was thought to determine completely that which followed. In such systems it appeared illegitimate to invoke final causes as a part of explanation. In recent years a profound change (134) has come from the study of systems which have characteristics of self-correction and are capable of predictive and adaptive responses. The reader will recognize that such systems closely simulate the characteristics of organisms, and in fact he will discover that they were anticipated by physiologists such as Claude Bernard, who as early as 1860 introduced the term *"milieu interne"* (26). The concept of internal environment and its consistency exerted a profound influence on physiologists, but not until Cannon's formulation (36), (37) of the concept of homeostatic mechanisms did the circular, self-corrective mechanism find explicit and official recognition in medicine. Today the majority of physicians and biologists utilize the concept of homeostasis as a scientific model to explain bodily processes (58).

A similar and concomitant development took place in the field of psychology and psychiatry. At the end of the nineteenth century and in the first decade of the twentieth, a radically new approach to psychiatry appeared on the horizon. Physiological psychology (165), (185) and classificatory psychiatry (91) were gradually being replaced by behaviorism (171), psychobiology (101), Gestalt psychology (89), and psychoanalysis (54). From concern with conscious statements the interest shifted to the study of unconscious features, the omission of statements, configuration, and background. Gradually the class-theoretical, Aristotelian approach (psychological types) was being replaced by the field theoretical approach (97) (psychological processes), and from static considerations of structure the focus shifted to considerations of process, until today reticulate chains of causation, circular systems, and social interaction are the main concern of most investigators.

Purpose of psychiatric systems. A combination of ideas derived from medicine, psychoanalysis, social work, psychology, and preventive medicine forms the background of the psychiatrist's theories of today. While the psychologist or sociologist searches for theories which would attempt to explain the multifarious aspects of human behavior, the psychiatrist is an engineer who searches for theories which would explain his therapeutic operations. At times, however, the psychiatrist has to proceed without a knowledge of complicated schemes. Then he acts intuitively, very much like a skilled administrator who, without being able to verbalize his plans beforehand, simply engages in certain operations which may or may not turn out to be successful. The knowledge which he possesses, therefore, remains unverbalized and implicit in his actions. Only after action has taken place is the administrator able to give a historical account of what has happened, and the psychiatrist is very much in the same position.

Now, in the twentieth century, the psychiatrist attempts to make up for this difficulty. On the one hand he tries to accumulate a body of information, and on the other he aspires to construct comprehensive theories (61), (93), (123) for the purpose of placing his intuitive and empirical approach on a more rational basis. While the scientific systems used in natural sciences and in philosophy were designed to give a satisfactory explanation about the information available at a given time, the contemporary psychiatric systems have a more restrictive character; they are designed to explain deviant behavior, change in behavior, and therapeutic operations rather than to encompass all the facts known about human behavior.

Position of the psychiatrist as observer. The building of systems to explain psychopathological events was undertaken by combining introspective knowledge with information obtained by observers looking at people from the outside. In psychiatric systems, therefore, we find that the position of the observer is not always clearly defined. At one time the system is designed to explain the observer's views from without, at another time it is used to explain the same system from within. Though concepts such as the "participant-observer" have been introduced to outline the unique and changing position of the psychiatrist, we shall point out in a later chapter that the theory of communication does show promise of solving this problem in a more satisfactory manner.

Structure and process. The problem of developing satisfactory scientific systems for psychiatric purposes has been further complicated by the circumstance that the description of behavioral processes in the past has unfailingly led to the development of psychological types. This particular feature of psychiatric theory can be blamed upon the fact that language refers to short-lasting processes as if these constituted an everlasting state. If a person, for example, makes such a statement as "Johnny is a liar," the data upon which the statement is based consist only of the fact that Johnny uttered some sentences which were not true. Because of this short burst of speech, he is given the title of liar, as if he were a liar twenty-four hours a day. He is placed in a category or type, and a single observation may provide the basis for such generalizations about his character features. On the one hand, the sentence "Johnny is a liar" conveys a description of a single event which actually took place; on the other hand this same sentence is a description of other potential behavior of Johnny, implying that he might lie again or that he is lying most of the time (73), (90), (117), (124).

Essentially these difficulties of description and typology are due to thinking in terms of structure rather than process. Both structure and process indicate methods by which the scientist handles information. In assessing the structure of things, an observer reduces numerous observations to a few statements which would indicate the relationship of those multiple factors at any one moment. The purpose of a structural statement, therefore, is to combine as many features as possible into one unit whereby changes in time are neglected. Conversely, in statements of process, the scientist tries to observe evolution in time. In order to accomplish this end he must make two, if not more, observations of a system of events over a period of time. The statement of process then combines into one unit these multiple factors which were observed at different dates. In order to describe human behavior, we use in our daily language expressions which refer to both structure and process; structural statements then denote the integration of features at a single instant, and can be expressed by purely spatial diagrams, while processal statements denote the continuing temporal integration. Varying his interest in structural or processal assessment of events, the scientist will choose the dimensions of his universe. Structural description permits the inclusion of many factors because changes in time are neglected; on the other hand, the consideration of processes demands a smaller delimitation because so many repeat observations have to be carried out (147).

Dimensions of psychiatric systems. However, the very same

interest in process which forces the scientist to limit the dimensions of his universe also makes him aware of the artificiality of his delineation. A brief review of the dimensions of scientific universes encountered by the psychiatrist might serve to illustrate this point.

The psychiatrist concerns himself with essentially five dimensions:

Dimension I. The unit of consideration is a part function of one individual: systemic systems, organ systems.

Dimension II. One human being as a whole is the unit: intrapersonal system of psychiatrist (54), (163).

Dimension III. The interaction of several individuals is the focus of interest: interpersonal systems (120), (160).

Dimension IV. The group is the center of the organization: anthropologist's systems of community, kinship, family, professional groups, and the like (14), (20), (92), (152).

Dimension V. The interaction of groups as focus of interest: societal systems as studied in economics, ecology, or political science (110), (111).

Nineteenth-century psychiatry was essentially interested in Dimension I, dealing with the part functions of one individual. As part functions in a psychological sense one may mention topics such as emotion, intellect, memory, mood, traits, habits, as well as all those headings referring to symptoms and syndromes. At the turn of the century the interest of psychiatrists shifted from Dimension I to Dimension II, and the intrapersonal structure became the center of attention. As time went on, towards the middle of the twentieth century, psychiatry became less concerned with structural models of the mind or the soul, and devoted more attention to the notions of process. In the last two decades, especially under the influence of the Washington School of Psychiatry (120), Dimension III, concerned with the interaction of individuals, has gained attention. At the moment the engineer's interest in problems of communication, the analyst's concern with transference and counter-transference, the sociologist's concern with group membership, document clearly the growing tendency of all disciplines to enlarge their previously restricted systems. For example, Dimension IV has already penetrated psychiatric thinking inasmuch as the structure of the family and other group relations have become foremost mental hygiene topics. And some aspects of socialized medicine definitely belong in Dimension V.

The system of Freud. At this point one ought to mention that Freud's greatest service to psychiatry was probably his introduction of the notion of process and the consideration of the individual as a whole. He met opposition and rattled the structurally minded psychiatrists of his time, but today psychiatry has finally adopted those notions of process which physicists and chemists had accepted a long time before. The system that Freud proposed for the explanation of intrapersonal events can be considered to be rather complete, inasmuch as it explains in a satisfactory manner most events within the universe of the psychiatrist. Freud's tripartite system (id, ego, and superego), however, still has some lineal characteristics, and events pertaining to the interaction of one individual with other persons and his participation in wider social events are not satisfactorily represented. As Ptolemy once postulated that our earth was the center of the astero-physical world, so Freud placed the intrapersonal processes at the center of all events. Today we must recognize that such a position is untenable. We will grant that for the understanding of intrapersonal processes Freud's model of the soul is still the most comprehensive system available. However, because of its lineal character and because of its relative isolation from other systems, it does not suffice to encompass all that happens between people. What we need today is systems which would embrace both events confined to the individual and events encompassing several people and larger groups (163).

Part and whole. The changing focus of the scientist's interest (33), (34), one minute concentrating on some small event occurring in a single cell, the next moment turning to the consideration of the organism in which this cell is located, raises a dialectical problem. The psychiatrist's operations make it necessary for him to focus his attention upon the individual as a whole, and information pertaining to part functions of the human being is left to fields such as physiological psychology, physiology, and pathology, while knowledge pertaining to the whole of society is willingly relegated to sociology, anthropology, and social psychology. Within the psychiatric systems proper, information pertaining to part functions of an individual is represented by such terms as "organic" or "somatic" and information referring to the larger societal systems by such terms as "environment." These expressions are global wastebaskets for events which are thought to fall beyond the limits of psychiatric concern. The existence of such events is noted, but attention is not devoted to any details. However, the psychiatrist cannot avoid shifting his focus of attention. At one instant he isolates a single event—let us say he observes a tic of the patient —and at the next instant he evaluates the tic in the perspective of all the information he possesses about the patient. Furthermore, he may at one instant consider the patient as an individual, and the next moment he may be concerned with the patient as a member of his family. Therefore he constantly switches the dimensions of his universe; this particular aspect we have termed the problem of "part and whole" (151).

During the last decade or so, awareness of the problem of part and whole has brought about a change of attitude. In recent years the psychiatrist, as well as all other social scientists, has realized that in order to understand the individual, information expressed in terms of various behavioral and societal systems has to be combined. This viewpoint is already gaining momentum but again, dialectical difficulties develop when scientists attempt to transfer information which is expressed in terms of a larger—e.g., societal—system to another system of a smaller dimension—e.g., the individual. Each system has its own language, and therefore it was necessary to carry along in scientific and interdisciplinary discussions the languages of these varied systems. Frequently the same events were labeled with a multiplicity of names, and these polyglot labels increased the existing confusion.

The need for a unified field theory, which would enable scientists to use one continuous set of terms and therefore eliminate the dialectical difficulties which develop with the shifting dimensions of the scientific universe, thus becomes quite apparent. And it is the hope of the authors to contribute towards a better understanding of the relationship of various scientific universes by proposing to consider within one system the communicative aspects of events (see Chapter 11) and thereby resolve the perennial discussion regarding the delineation of such entities as society, group, individual, organ, and cells.

Variables in psychiatric systems. If in the last few pages we have been concerned with the most abstract principles which govern psychiatric thinking, we now shall descend the ladder of complexity and be concerned with the variables which govern psychiatric thinking. Let us first inspect the topics which psychiatrists write and talk about, and derive from these the ingredients or elements which make up the psychiatric systems. Inasmuch as Murphy (121), Nicole (122), and Janet (83), (84) have excellent reviews of the varied approaches, viewpoints, and systems which psychiatrists use, we shall refrain from repeating that which is well known. The reader who is familiar with this source material will understand that the subject matter of psychiatry can be conveniently divided into five large groups. These groupings, which for brevity's sake we shall refer to as topics, are an expression not only of observed events, but also of the psychiatrist's ways of managing the information he has acquired. His focus, his attitudes, and his viewpoints are revealed in the slants taken in his publications and lectures. These slants not only differentiate the psychiatrists from each other, but they also establish fashion trends and procedure for future generations. Up to now, when psychiatrists have expressed a scientific opinion, they have tended to maximize one or more of the following aspects:

First, we find that the psychiatrist operates with genetically determined variables which are statements of varied purpose and potentiality in human beings. These are subsumed under such topics as heredity, constitution, and homeostasis, and they are thought to be beyond the control of any individual. Such a predeterministic outlook forces the psychiatrist into a position of maximizing *structurally organic determinants.*

Second, the psychiatrist operates with biologically determined variables which are statements about the hypothetical and immediate causes of overt behavior in human beings. The individual is thought to be incapable of changing the forces which are subsumed under headings such as instincts, drives, needs, and the "id." However, such a view, which maximizes the *animalistic forces* in the human being, assumes that there are other forces which can counteract, reinforce, or alienate the effect of these primitive urges.

Third, the psychiatrist assumes the existence of forces which are opposed to the animalistic tendencies of the human being. The psychiatrist believes that these learned, complex, and experientially determined features exert a stabilizing influence which opposes the unstable and often asocial animalistic forces inherent in human beings. These *humanistic features* have been called attitudes, interests, aspirations, will power, reason, "ego ideal," or "superego."

Fourth, the psychiatrist uses variables which are thought to implement the various needs of the individual. These variables are summarized under such headings as emotions, feelings, moods, memory, abilities, talents, instrumental actions, responses, implementations, or the "ego." These forces are thought to implement carnal and spiritual—that is, animalistic and humanistic—motivations of the individual. Psychiatrists who maximize these variables are essentially concerned with *effector determinants.*

Fifth, there are all those realistically and culturally determined variables which are dictated by the surroundings. These *environmental determinants,* including all social and economic factors, the psychiatrist uses as a background against which he explains some of the events which cannot be explained in any other terms.

The hodgepodge of variables appearing in psychiatric systems has been introduced by a multiplicity of factors: one source being history and tradition, another the scientific disciplines from which the information derived, and a third the practical operations of the psychiatrist. The psychiatrist's thinking, by and large, circles around psychological and philosophical considerations of biological events; he is concerned with life and death, with the purpose of things, with limitations of the human being, with determinism of human behavior, with the mastery of biological functions, and the like. Thus we find that his information has been borrowed from natural sciences, biology, the humanities, and religion; rationally, however, the psychiatric systems really make little sense; they are primarily anthropological and historical museums of philosophical, psychological, and religious considerations of past centuries.

Processes described in psychiatric systems. Nor do we find more consistency if we attempt to specify the life processes with which the psychiatrist is concerned. It will not be a surprise to the reader to find that the psychiatrist's views consist of a composite mixture of biological, psychological, and social considerations; the common denominator of these diverse views is found in the fact that the human being is a biological organism, characterized by a life cycle and by purposive behavior. In pursuing his study of the life cycle of organisms, the psychiatrist developed a set of variables which run along a scale ranging from *progression* to *regression*. Progression would denote the development of inherent potentialities of the organism until optimal functioning has been attained, while regression would include all those processes which lead to ultimate decay. Growth, learning, conditioning, maturation, and integration would be examples of progressive processes, while headings such as decline, deterioration, senescence would illustrate regressive processes. It is interesting to note that part of Freud's psychological system is built on this notion of progression-regression, and that in addition to considering an over-all trend, he also introduced the notion of short-lasting regressional periods within a major progressional cycle. Today it is widely accepted that at times of stress the individual tends to regress by resorting again to implementations and means of gratification which were used in an earlier developmental period. It seems as if the concepts of progression and regression were the psychiatric version of the nineteenth-century concern with evolution and the twentieth-century interest in problems of periodicity.

Psychiatrists have been deeply influenced by the physiologists' views of homeostasis and by all those concepts referring to steady-state mechanisms. And after accepting these modern biological concepts the psychiatrist had to develop psychological concepts which in some way would be equivalent to the views prevailing in other natural sciences. Therefore we are not surprised to find that the psychiatrist developed psychological concepts which are direct analogies to the physical processes of metabolism, storage of energy, and elimination of waste products. Freud's concepts of orality and anality and the further refinements introduced later (1), (52) were designed to adapt psychological processes to conform to concepts of physiology. In some ways violence was done to the nature of psychological events by treating them as if they were chemical or physical events. Thus a psychoanalyst talks about incorporation, retention, and elimination, using physiological analogies of food intake and digestion to explain such highly complicated mechanisms as conditioning, retention of sensory impressions, or volitional acts. In using such analogies psychoanalysts followed the nineteenth-century fashion of studying body functions by dissecting organs and considering systems separately as if they existed in isolation from other functions. It is well to remember that a brain is not at all the same thing at autopsy as it is when the central nervous system is a part of a living organism. And it is also well to remember that the baby already reacts as a whole organism in which all functions are subordinated to the foremost task at any given moment. Today most scientists look askance at attempts to split the organism into part functions, and the old attempts to dissect the individual psychologically have fortunately been abandoned.

The physical problems of maintenance and steady state and other psychological analogies are probably responsible for the psychiatrist's concern with the problem of *interference*. Volumes have been written on the nature of aggression and whether aggressive acts are the outgrowth of a primary instinct or are responses to outside interference (48). Be that as it may, the existence of interference cannot be denied. We all know that the organism is equipped to respond in various ways to threatening events. Upon perception of a strange or threatening stimulus, the organism reacts with alarm. Muscular, vascular, psychological, and chemical processes are set in motion which enable the organism to proceed with action and to sustain maximum effort for a limited period of time (146), (148). Depending upon the situation, the reaction of the alarmed individual can be described as anger, fear, or anxiety. If anger develops, the alarm reaction will be used for fighting; if fear develops, for running away and avoidance; if both types of action are prevented, anxiety will develop. Shame, guilt, and depression denote the response of the individual to alarm in response to stimuli which arise within the individual himself.

Reactions to interfering stimuli from without or within can sometimes assume emergency proportions which disrupt not only the functioning of a particular individual, but also of the group of which he is a member. Acute "nervous breakdowns," tension states, and the phenomena of anger, fear, anxiety, shame, guilt, and depression are the principle concerns of the psychiatrist (138). These terms designate essentially symptoms which develop when a breakdown in the system of communication of the patient occurs. However, most psychiatric theories attempt to explain these phenomena in terms of the individual only. They do not include other persons or the social matrix in which an individual lives, and in which these events occur. This is the most outstanding weakness of present-day psychiatric theory.

Likewise, the tendency to dissect the functioning of individuals into *mechanisms* is a great weakness of theoretical psychiatry. When the psychiatrist refers to identification, projection, sublimation, reaction formation, and so on, he is making statements about his own focus of attention rather than explaining what goes on in another individual. These mechanisms do not constitute separable units of behavior which could legitimately be used as explanations of what is happening; rather, the reference to one of these mechanisms is an explanation indicating some features of the momentary focus of the psychiatrist's perceptions. If the reader will take the trouble to think through what is meant by one of these "mechanisms," he soon will discover that in order to explain and understand any one of them, all the other mechanisms are also needed. The word "mechanism" is, in fact, a misnomer. "Projection," "identification," and so on, are elements in the functioning of a total individual as perceived and dissected by another individual (the scientist). If these elements were represented in a diagram, the diagram would not be comparable to a block diagram of existing parts within the single individual; rather, it would be a *flow chart* in which the units represent "functions" or "processes." Furthermore, this flow chart would represent not one individual but two persons in interaction.

General postulates of psychiatric theories. In order to further understand the nature of psychiatric theories of our time we shall attempt to trace all psychiatric concepts to five premises. The first is related to the concept of normality and pathology, the second to the concept of polarity, and the third to the constant search for causes; the fourth is the psychiatrist's tendency to relate momentary behavior to a spectrum of behavior over a longer period of time, and the fifth is related to the psychiatrist's relativistic attitudes. Though it would be absurd to pretend that these are the only premises which psychiatrists use, nonetheless it seems as if all statements of psychiatrists, especially those which qualify human behavior, have some features in common. The data from which these premises were derived can be found in any textbook of psychiatry and can be verified in any lecture given by a psychiatrist.

To arrange scientific data in an orderly manner the psychiatrist uses as one of his principles the concept of *pathology*. Implicitly, therefore, he classifies the phenomena which he observes in terms of deviation from the norm. In this context the concept of pathology has a statistical meaning denoting preoccupation with infrequent events which because of their rare occurrence are labeled pathological.

In a second context pathology may also be defined as a concept which denotes deviation from the ideal, desirable, or optimal state of functioning regardless of statistical frequency. This latter meaning derives from medical usage. The psychiatrist who by training and vocation is a physician, unconsciously —and sometimes consciously—evaluates a patient in terms of actual functioning, both physical and mental; he then compares his findings to the level which the patient might achieve under optimal circumstances. Medical or psychiatric findings which deviate markedly from this optimum are then labeled pathological.

A third meaning of the concept of pathology is found when the psychiatrist compares the symptoms and signs of his patients with those of known and established disease entities; this process of matching individual findings with established pathology is used in diagnostic procedures.

The psychological, personality, and psychopathological systems used by psychiatrists are all based essentially upon the concept of disordered function or pathology. But inasmuch as psychiatrists themselves do not possess a sufficiently clear notion of normality, the question may be raised whether the concept of the norm is not opposed and in contradiction to the concept of individual adjustment and adaptation. Be that as it may, some of the confusion existing in psychiatry today is clearly related to the improper use of a rather nebulous concept of normality. In order to avoid the difficulties which arise in the traditional classification of psychopathological events, some psychiatrists have introduced the notion that each individual is unique, so that the concept of normality or deviation cannot be applied, and that instead the concept of internal consistency should be used. If this were completely true, however, training in psychiatry and psychotherapy would be futile because one would have to assume, each case being so different from the next one, that no generalizations could be made. The fact that psychiatrists can be trained, however, speaks to the contrary (11). Therefore we must assume that all therapists operate with some concept of normality which allows them to make generalizations, even if this is vehemently denied. Perhaps we have to think of normality on a higher level of abstraction than is commonly accepted. One can state with certainty that the biological and psychological similarities of man are greater than his differences, and that the minimum physiological and psychological requirements compatible with health and the limits of maximal human efforts are well known. Within this range, then, some generalizations can be made and within this context predictions regarding human behavior are safe.

In order to understand the psychiatrist's thinking one must bear in mind that his daily activities revolve around mental abnormalities and that concern with the psychological norm falls into the periphery of his endeavors. Following the diagnostic operations of psychiatrists, for example, a patient is labeled normal only in the absence of "pathological" features. The diagnosis of normality is made by exclusion, and if a psychiatrist can label a feature it is by implication pathological and undesirable. Therefore anything that is called by a name is implicitly abnormal, and in the existing psychiatric nomenclature of diagnoses, syndromes, symptoms, patterns, mechanisms, habits, and the like, this procedure is clearly revealed. Since the psychiatrist's attention is focused upon deviation, and since he has little or no training in normal psychology, he tends to construct a hypothetical norm by averaging the exact opposite of those features he sees in his patients. In therapy the assumption of a norm so constructed works very satisfactorily. Indirectly and implicitly, the psychiatrist exerts considerable pressure upon patients to focus upon their abnormal features. The result of such isolation of abnormal features against a hypothetical background of normality and health gives psychotherapy aim and direction. It might suffice to mention here such concepts as maturity and regression, the pleasure principle and the reality principle, to illustrate our case.

The nature of pathology implies the existence of a concept of health, and all medical and psychiatric thinking is geared toward helping the patient achieve health. Mental health is obviously defined in terms of the culture in which the patient and the therapist live. The concept of health can be viewed as a structural assumption describing a series of conditions pertinent to processes which prolong the optimal functioning of an individual. The concept of disease, in contrast, denotes deviation from optimal functioning through the introduction of a number of reversible or irreversible processes. Inasmuch as health is defined in each culture in terms of those physical and mental processes which seem to be desirable to the system in power, the American concept of health can be derived from that which will be said about the American culture as a whole. To be able to compete and to successfully grasp the opportunity which equality provides for the individual defines the essential meaning of living in America. In order to do these things, an American citizen must be strong, self-reliant, independent, free of physical disease, able to get along in a group, ready to adapt to emergencies, capable of caring for children and the family, and not a public liability. The healthy individual is expected to use his power for his own benefit with restraint and wisdom.

The concept of health is very popular in America. There are the United States Public Health Service, the departments of health of states, counties, and communities, and the various leagues for fighting specific diseases and for the rehabilitation of invalids. Every citizen is aware that cleanliness and hygiene are necessary concerns of successful living, and early training at home is fortified by later teaching in school; the child learns the idea that bodily and dental care, nutrition, and fresh air are all necessary conditions for successfully carrying on competitive striving. In this atmosphere of hygiene, psychotherapy can of course thrive, and the public expects from a psychotherapeutic movement more or less the same results as it expects from dental care. A program of prevention, a set of formulas to cope with emergencies, general directions for ordinary living and institutional facilities for those who cannot fit into the group are expected from psychiatry.

It is not surprising, therefore, to see that in all countries medical and psychiatric theories are influenced by the efforts of therapists to bring about health. Those who are pure scientists and not therapists develop theories of human behavior which are not suitable for understanding deranged functions in therapeutic operations. In contrast, the person whose motivation is to help the sick develops concepts of pathology which are subservient to the methods of treatment. When the psychiatrist talks about abnormal behavior, it sometimes appears to a neutral observer that the psychiatrist is a pure scientist: his scope and purpose seem limited to the acquisition of information as a goal in itself. This, however, is only half the truth, because the psychiatrist wants to use the information in certain operations. These two facets of the psychiatrist—the scientific and the manipulative—have always puzzled observers who come from the pure sciences, and most of the criticism directed at psychiatry derives from a misunderstanding of the psychiatrist's purpose.

The construction of a hypothetical norm in the mind of the psychiatrist or, on the other hand, the declaration that a feature is abnormal and must be remedied, brings out another scientific concept—namely, that of *polarity*. Bipolar variables such as intelligent or stupid, conscious or unconscious, mature or immature, real or imagined, gratified or frustrated, and the like, are an expression of linear systems of thinking, in which two poles indicate two extremes with the middle being the norm; sometimes one of the poles denotes deviation and the other the norm. For example, the terms "abstainer" and "alcoholic" denote two extremes, whereas "temperate" would indicate the norm; on the other hand, the term "balanced" would indicate norm, and "unbalanced" the pathological deviation.

In all systems of psychiatry polar concepts are widely used, and it is well to remember that medicine is based upon the dichotomy of health and disease. Both the principle of pathology and the principle of polarity are subservient to the fact that the occupation of healing is unthinkable without some value judgments about health and disease. Inasmuch as the psychiatrist's activity is primarily devoted to the improvement of mental health rather than to the collection of information, he must, of necessity, divide events into those which are useful and those which are not. Codes of ethics bearing upon human conduct are seldom derived from any scientific accumulation of information but are rather the result of pressure from religious, political, and other groups which prescribe some standard of human behavior.

Sickness is culturally defined, and likewise society provides an institutional solution for those who are sick. In all cultures there are explanations of sickness; in our culture the explanation is the province of physicians who search for the causes responsible for the pathology. The theories of *causality* which psychiatrists of the past have developed have usually been dominated either by superstition or by physiological and mechanistic thinking. In an attempt to explain the causes of mental illness, various fashion trends, viewing mental disease as the result of witchcraft or as the result of bacterial invasion, have had their day. In the last hundred years, the medical concept of etiology which consisted in searching for the immediate causes of a disease or of a deranged function has dominated psychiatry at large. Physicians tended to ask the question "why," which essentially derived from Aristotelian systems of thinking, rather than to raise the question "how," which derived from modern field-theoretical approaches. In the Aristotelian or class-theoretical approach, things were classified in categories; the reader is but too familiar with Kraepelin's classificatory system of psychiatry (91) to require further exemplification. The answer to the question "why," then, consisted of searching for a cause which would explain the existence of such a class of diseases. In contrast, the field-theoretical approach is concerned with the functional relations between a system of events and the field in which they occur; applied to human behavior it would mean concern with the relationship of an individual and his environment. While the class-theoretical approach presupposes lineal, branching, or converging systems or chains of causation, the field-theoretical approach is concerned with circular systems and self-regulatory mechanisms (97), (180).

In the modern approach one asks how something operates within a given system, while in the past one was concerned with the question of why such a system came into existence. In psychiatry ancient thinking still is strongly represented. For example, there exists the belief that if one could find that one "Factor X" which is responsible for a given nosological entity such as schizophrenia, one could cure such a condition. The fallacy of such argument is obvious. Raising the question of the cause of schizophrenia presupposes that certain behavioral features can be classified, isolated, and localized and that the hypothetical cause can be likewise isolated and related to the disease entity. In such reasoning, the organism is not considered as a whole but is split up in part functions. Likewise, in psychotherapy, there exists still the tendency to make single events such as traumatic childhood experiences responsible for later behavior. Causal and lineal thinking are also revealed in fashion trends of psychoanalysis, varying from the "primal scene" over the "castration complex" to "repressed aggression." This strong nineteenth-century orientation of psychiatric theory is likely to be replaced in time by more modern views. These hold that whenever one factor changes, all the other factors likewise must undergo change; therefore in observing steady-state mechanisms of the organism, for example in the form of stabilized behavior patterns, it is usually impossible to isolate single causes which can be made directly responsible for the present picture. The most that can be done is to specify the conditions which existed previously and those which exist now, without knowing too much about the relation of multiple causes and multiple effects. The modern psychiatrist's theoretical views have to take care of a multitude of facts; the psychiatrist has to realize that he himself, and also the individual he is studying, are but minimal parts of larger superpersonal systems and that the theories of causality which the psychiatrist establishes are usually valid only within the framework of very narrow considerations, special situations, and limited delineations of the scientific universe.

The psychiatrist's answer to questions bearing upon the cause of mental conditions is ultimately connected with his tendency to isolate one behavioral event and to view it against the whole *background of information* he possesses about an individual. The psychiatrist who sees a patient under interview conditions and for a short period of time does not think of the patient in terms of his momentary observations alone. In order to proceed with therapy, the psychiatrist wishes to gain an understanding of the patient's personality as a whole; this means that he attempts to construct within his own mind a small-scale model of the patient's entire life and attempts to place present observations of the patient's actions within this larger framework. For example, if the patient is smoking a cigarette, the psychiatrist would want to inquire when the patient smoked his first cigarette, and he will be curious to know whether the patient's mother had given him a lollipop when adults were smoking in the living room; he might even consider the time when the bottle or breast satisfied the oral needs of the patient. Thus the psychiatrist views a single act at the present time with a background of the inferred over-all behavior of the patient. At this point it is well to remember that a single act or series of actions can be observed by anybody who is present, but that the over-all behavior, over the past twenty years, for example, exists only in the form of information which condenses into one moment the serial happenings over a period of time. In psychiatric theories of causality a single outside event is equated with a spectrum of information in the mind of the observer. In theories of physics two outside events are connected with a spectrum of information present in the mind of the observer. In psychiatry we are thus faced with the problem of considering a part with the background of a whole. The part is defined by our biological limitations as human beings—that is, our machinery for the reception and transmission of messages; the whole is defined by our ability to conceptualize. We call the problem dialectical essentially because it is related to the peculiarities of the observer, rather than being structured by the nature of observed events (151).

Another difficulty of the psychiatrist in establishing valid theories of causation involves his particular personality and the role in which he governs a social situation. A verbal statement perceived by an observer can be interpreted in different ways. For example, a compulsive or legalistic mind might confine itself to purely syntactical or semantic interpretations, omitting all pragmatic considerations. In contrast, the psychologically oriented person will listen to the same statement in an attempt to detect the implied values of the speaker. A politically minded person with common sense will in turn interpret the statement as an expression of the feeling of the population at large and without particular consideration of the individual who makes the statement. Thus the legalistic mind acts primarily as an observer, the psychologically minded person as a participant, and the politically minded person, while he may pretend to participate, is in reality manipulating, campaigning, and observing the effects of his actions. The psychiatrist uses all three attitudes for purposes of understanding and carrying out therapy; in his therapeutic role, not only does he change his position as participant and observer, but he also switches the levels of abstraction in emitting and receiving messages. For example, when the psychiatrist uses a term like "castration," several meanings are conveyed. First, the literal meaning of an actual physical injury to the genital region; second, an injury to all those symbols which stand for genitalia; third, the restriction of freedom and independence which is necessary for the preliminary explorations preceding the use of genitalia; and last, on the highest level of abstraction, he may use "castration" to refer to any forced relinquishment of ideas or rights which in some remote way may influence genital functioning. Psychiatric variables are thus characterized by the fact that they pertain simultaneously to different levels of abstraction, and only prolonged contact with the psychiatric fraternity enables a stranger to learn all the cues which indicate the particular level of abstraction at which the message is to be interpreted.

The multiple meaning of the psychiatric vocabulary is extremely useful in therapy. It enables the psychiatrist to proceed from more restricted to more inclusive considerations, and it increases the awareness of the patient with regard to his own and other people's actions; therefore it exerts an integrative influence upon the patient. However, it is quite clear that such elastic and multiple meanings of words do not lend themselves to precise definition and therefore to the development of theories of causality.

This brings us to the last basic aspect of psychiatric thinking, the psychiatrist's *relativism*. The psychiatrist's tolerance and permissiveness in therapy necessitates that he abstain from overt value judgments. However, this position is somehow untenable outside of the therapeutic situation if one considers that there are things, methods, and approaches which are more suitable than others for a given purpose. For example, we all know that there are tires which last longer than others, that there are agricultural procedures which produce better milk, and that there are social techniques and schemes which give more satisfaction to the majority of people than others. And there is hardly anybody who would question the statement that war, utter destruction, and famine are worse than peace, constructive ways of living, and assurance of satisfactory standards of living. Thus there is no doubt that there are methods which are better than others; but in spite of this evidence the psychiatrist generally refrains from making judgments, acting strictly as a historian. He confines himself to that which has happened, and he helps the patient to draw necessary conclusions from events of the past; he holds to the view that any step to be undertaken in the future is as good as any other if it works out well. The fact that one approach is successful for a single individual does not necessarily mean that the scheme as such is superior to any other; all that it means is that within a given set of restricted circumstances a particular scheme has turned out to be successful.

This pragmatic relativism of the psychiatrist and his waiving of absolute values seem to be an expression of our time. People seem to have lost the ability to make theoretical decisions which would promote a consistent viewpoint. Instead they make pragmatic choices in terms of specified goals, and we shall show later that the American premise of equality has largely contributed to the widespread acceptance of such pragmatism.

The confusion between theoretical and pragmatic equality was perceived by Abraham Lincoln, who said, "I think the authors of the Declaration of Independence intended to include all men, but they did not intend to declare all men equal in all respects."

At the present time psychiatry and the American public at large seem to hold the view that all people are born with similar potentialities, and that the differences observed are primarily due to variations in environment, opportunity, and achievement. Be that as it may, within the framework of relativism and pragmatism, theory is laid aside when immediate application in action is not possible. The American psychiatrist strives more for therapeutic success than for an understanding of the therapeutic processes.

It goes without saying that any scientific theory is man-made; the scientists who formulate it live in a given country at a given time, and are subject to the influence of their contemporaries. Any scientific theory therefore reflects in some way the culture in which it was created. The system of cues and clues which the given culture provides to enable people to understand each other is necessarily used by the theorist in forming and stating his theory; and therefore the theory can only be fully understood after this system of cues has been studied.

Moreover, the culture enters again into the formation of psychiatric theory because the goals of psychiatry are culturally determined; the concepts and evaluation of health and disease which determine the operations (and therefore the viewpoints) of psychiatrists differ from culture to culture.

So far we have pointed out some of the difficulties existing in the theory and practice of psychiatry. We have called attention to the fact that the basic requirements for the construction of a psychiatric system are that it be circular, that it have the characteristics of self-correction, that it satisfactorily solve the problem of part and whole function, and that it clearly define the position of the observer and therefore state the influence of the observer upon that which is observed and vice versa. In subsequent paragraphs we shall explain that these characteristics are fulfilled by conceiving and explaining psychiatric events in terms of a system of communication. We shall discuss how such a system facilitates the understanding of psychiatric events and the formulation of therapeutic procedures, and how it also bridges the gap between psychiatry and other fields of social science.

DISTURBANCES OF COMMUNICATION AND PSYCHOTHERAPY

Psychopathology is defined in terms of disturbances of communication. This statement may come as a surprise, but if the reader cares to open a textbook on psychiatry and to read about the manic-depressive or the schizophrenic psychosis, for example, he is likely to find terms such as "illusions," "delusions," "hallucinations," "flight of ideas," "disassociation," "mental retardation," "elation," "withdrawal," and many others, which refer specifically to disturbances of communication; they imply either that perception is distorted or that expression—that is, transmission—is unintelligible.

Psychiatrists who devote their time to psychotherapy believe that the rehabilitation of patients suffering from psychopathology can only be carried out within the context of a social situation; they think that contact with human beings is a therapeutic necessity. If one attempts to analyze the events which take place in a social situation, the interaction between patient and doctor, and the efforts directed at influencing the patient by means of psychotherapy, one must arrive at the conclusion that these events fall into the realm of communication. Therefore one can state with certainty that the therapeutically effective agents contained in psychotherapy are to be found in communication.

In attempting to isolate and narrow down those communicative processes which seem to have a therapeutic effect we find that the existing formulations do not do justice to the processes of communication, although concepts such as "transference," "countertransference," "catharsis," and "free association" implicitly refer to the communicative aspects of psychoanalytic procedures. These terms were designed to fit into systems which were oriented around the individual as an isolated entity rather than around his functions as a social being. Therefore it is not surprising to discover that while all therapists actually attempt to improve the means of communication of their patients, when they talk about these events, they mention only implicitly the processes of communication.

The scant information pertaining to communication stands in sharp contrast to the numerous publications which attempt to explain what happens in the minds of individuals. Inasmuch as the theoretical schemes were geared to the isolated consideration of single human beings, no provision was made for the inclusion of the surroundings or of the social relations of a person. Today, therefore, it has become necessary to widen the concepts which deal with personality structure, to include hypotheses which would encompass all the people who interact in both therapeutic and social situations. When we enlarge our psychiatric considerations to embrace the wider networks of communication, we cease to limit ourselves to the boundaries of one individual. We are now interested, rather, in tracing incoming and outgoing messages in time and space to their source and destination.

The network of communication, therefore, is going to define our psychiatric universe. The origin and destination of messages may be found within the same organism; then we are dealing with an intrapersonal network. If the message originates in one person and is perceived by another, we are dealing with an interpersonal network. If an individual has the function of messenger, then both the origin and destination lie outside that particular organism. Therefore, in order to understand a communication system, and especially the disturbances of communication arising in such a system, the attention of the psychiatrist has to focus on the social situation; the focus of interaction will then be the interaction of people, the influence of mass communication upon the individual, and the shaping of the larger and more complex superpersonal systems through the summation of actions of single individuals (147).

Viewing psychotherapy primarily as an attempt at improving the communication of the patient within himself and with others raises a question as to the conditions which are necessary to bring about such improvement (60). We have mentioned before that a stranger is in a specially favorable position to make value statements about people whom he has observed. The tourist, when he tries to engage in a conversation with people of a foreign country, has to explore their system of communication. He may have learned the foreign language at home, but missing the many associations which are necessary for a meaningful interpretation of the messages received from others, he is at a loss to understand what is going on and especially to understand the emotional shadings of human relationships. This experience is familiar to the American who may visit England. He hears approximately the same language, but in no way does he understand the subtle shadings of behavior and expression of the Englishman until he has mastered, through a long series of experiences, the necessary cues which enable him to interpret the Englishman's messages correctly.

The general principle which underlies these observations may be stated as follows: When all participants adhere to the same system of communication, a spontaneous give-and-take develops, because implicitly these participants know how to communicate, although explicitly they are frequently unable to formulate their methods of communication. In contrast, when people use different systems of communication they must first acquire explicit information about their own and the other person's ways of communication before a satisfactory exchange can take place.

The psychiatrist who wishes to converse with a hebephrenic patient, therefore, is in very much the same position as a tourist who travels in a foreign country and is unfamiliar with the language. He has to explore the particular communication system which the patient uses in order to understand the content of the message, a task which frequently involves the insurmountable job of decoding the symbolic system of the patient. Therefore one might assume that in any therapeutic procedure where understanding between persons is a guiding mode of operation, differences between patient and therapist are essential if the patient is to make favorable progress. Specifically, it seems that the important differences are differences in the communication system of the two persons and that the progress of therapy is related to the patient's experience, conscious or unconscious, of communicating with another individual—the therapist— whose values and communication system are different from his own.

The central problem of psychotherapy may now be restated as follows: How does it happen that in the interchange of messages between two persons with differing systems of codification and evaluation, a change occurs in the system of codification and evaluation of either one or both persons? This problem touches on the paradox that, at a given instant, an individual can only emit or receive messages structured appropriately for his communication system as it exists at that moment. All other messages must be supposed to remain either unperceived, unintelligible, or misunderstood. In interaction, when an individual is actually participating in person-to-person communication, it is possible for him to perceive that messages have remained misunderstood, and that information is missing. In situations where messages are conveyed by the printed word, such detection of omission is difficult if not impossible.

The difference between communication in person-to-person contact and communication through the printed word is in part responsible for the discrepancy between psychiatric theory and therapeutic practice. It is difficult to evoke through a written message the same impression as that conveyed through word of mouth in personal contact, and this difficulty is related to the characteristics of language. Inasmuch as communication has to be used to write about communication, we find ourselves very much in the same position as the man who attempts to pull himself up by his bootstraps. However, there exist solutions to this puzzle. The novelist, for example, who is aware of these snags, writes about communication by re-enacting on paper a situation involving human relations and leaves that which is said about communication implicit. He, as an artist, sets the stage; he introduces us to the performers, he engages them in action, and he makes us, the readers, feel as if we were right there, participating as a spectator, on the scene of action. And after reading the last page we close the book with the feeling that a lot of things have happened to us in the span of time that it took us to devour page after page of the plot. Our gratitude and admiration, or hatred and condemnation, will acknowledge the artist's attempts to bring life into words and sentences.

But as scientists we cannot quite react to the type of presentation used by the artist. One must remember that whenever a novelist presents a series of events, he counts on producing a somewhat kinesthetic impression upon the reader; in these successive impressions which are received when reading a book from beginning to end, the novelist transmits to us that which, through the unidimensionality of language, is lost in scientific writing. In prose and poetry, sensory impressions and more composite emotional states are elicited in the reader implicitly through the effects of printed messages, spaced in time. Through skillful handling of sequences and contrasts, close-ups and panoramic views, focus and fadeout, the artist overcomes the unidimensionality of language.

The dilemma that the psychiatrist is faced with is related to the unidimensionality of language. In describing an event which took place between people he can be explicit with regard to what occurred and leave the underlying principles implicit. In this case, and assuming that the man is gifted in accurate description, he will put on paper whatever impresses him most. This arbitrary but unavoidable procedure is necessary because the wealth of simultaneous impressions must be expressed successively. By the time the observer gets around to writing down whatever he perceived, new and therefore more urgent sensory impressions have displaced the old ones, and most of what was perceived is lost.

An alternate solution of the psychiatrist is to abstract and condense his observations before writing them down; selectivity, therefore, becomes an unavoidable issue. Proceeding in such a manner, the observer will tend to become explicit about principles involved in a social event. But whenever a psychiatrist becomes explicit about principles, he is traveling on a one-way street. He may save time, but he pays a price, inasmuch as reconstruction of original events from inferred principles is impossible. In order to overcome this limitation, the psychiatrist, when discussing principles, tends to refer back to the original events; in practice this is achieved by citing an illustrative case. Literary productions of psychiatrists are characterized by this mixture of principles and case reports. But even then, a reader who was not present when the original event happened may not understand the written report because the selectivity of the reporter may have omitted the pertinent data to which the principles apply. To this objection the psychiatrist tends to reply that for real understanding a person must become a participant in a social situation; events experienced in common can then be used as a basis for further discussion of principles. The limitations of this procedure are obvious; only a selected few can participate in any one situation, and a cumulative body of knowledge is difficult to compile on such a basis.

Some psychiatrists even maintain that psychiatry and psychotherapy can only be taught through person-to-person contact; they believe that exposure to mass communication through books and lectures is completely ineffectual. Though there is a great deal of truth in this statement, quite obviously it does not correspond to the reality situation. Let us grant that the "when" and "how much" of the art of therapy can only be learned through personal experience, and that each individual has to develop his own skill. The "what" and the "where," however, are aspects of therapy which fall into the realm of science, and with regard to these aspects a cumulative body of scientific knowledge can be compiled.

The "when" and "how much" of the art of therapy depends upon a person's ability to master a variety of systems of communication as they are encountered in disturbed patients. Here it is not so much the knowledge of these systems that matters, but rather the ability to communicate within such systems as they are set up by the patient. To go back to our analogy about the traveler, the psychiatrist is here required to communicate with the spontaneity of the child or of the native. In contrast, the "what" and the "where" of therapy are expressions of explicit knowledge about these systems. When thinking, talking, or writing about patients, the psychiatrist is required to act as if he were a traveler who is reporting his experiences while traveling abroad; these experiences, by and large, are expressions of the clash of different systems of communication and therefore of implementation.

Disturbances of communication are understood best by a participant-observer attitude (160), which enables the psychiatrist to decide whether or not a person is suffering from disturbances of communication, and if so, to initiate the necessary processes for their correction. In the course of an initial interview we would proceed about as follows: First we would ascertain whether the patient is aware of rules, roles, and the label of social situations, and whether he is able to evaluate correctly the context of his communication system.

In a second step we would observe whether or not the focus of the patient corresponds to the network of communication in which he is actually participating. We would search for disturbances in the intrapersonal network, which may appear in the form of disturbances in the perception of external stimuli (exteroception), in the perception of internal stimuli (proprioception), in central operations with information at hand (codification-evaluation), in the transmission of messages from the center to other parts of the body (propriotransmission), or in the transmission of messages to the outside world (exterotransmission). We would ascertain how a person functions within an interpersonal network and as a member of group and cultural networks. The functioning of a patient in an interpersonal situation can only be ascertained if the psychiatrist exposes himself to the impact of the messages of the patient, and once he has received these, if he watches the impact of his own communications upon the patient. In such a circular system the observation of feedback operations enables the psychiatrist to assess the patient's ability or inability to correct messages received and sent, which correction necessitates the patient's observation of his impact upon others, and of others upon himself.

It goes without saying that the psychiatrist, as a physician, will also pay attention to the quantitative aspects of communication; the intensity of the stimuli with respect to overstimulation or understimulation and all the other aspects of metabolism of the organism are here of interest.

In a fourth step, we would consider the semantic problems of communication which are concerned with the precision with which a patient's messages transmit the desired meaning. The linguistic aspects, the mastery of symbolic systems, and the whole problem of higher learning are here of relevance.

In a last step we then will gauge the effectiveness with which the patient's messages influence the conduct of other persons in a desirable or undesirable way. Mastery of communication would mean that the desired effect can be achieved and that this effect upon others will be to the patient's benefit; and that if it is to the patient's benefit, it will by and large benefit others with whom he is in contact.

Such a formulation obviously raises the question of the influence of the psychiatrist within a system of communication and of the validity of his conclusions. As a result of participation in the system—and non-participation is impossible—the patient's behavior is going to be influenced by the psychiatrist, and vice versa. Not only may the patient get better or worse while we explore him for the first time, but our own disturbances of communication may obscure our assessment of the patient. We are never quite secure in what we are doing, and only a check by another person, either an outsider or the patient himself, will enable us to gauge the effect of our own actions. The ability to mutually correct the meaning of messages and to mutually influence each other's behavior to each other's satisfaction is the result of successful communication. This is the only criterion we possess, and if we achieve such a state, it indicates mental health.

If the ability to communicate successfully becomes synonymous with being mentally healthy, we are well aware of the fact that such a definition is a relativistic one; but it is obvious that people are mentally healthy only when their means of communication permit them to manage their surroundings successfully. Either when the means of communication are not available and breakdown occurs, or when people are transplanted to surroundings which use a different system of communication, these people become temporarily or permanently maladjusted. Inasmuch as no surroundings are ever stable, we have to continually correct our information; knowledge obtained under a given set of circumstances or in one type of social situation has to be checked in the context of other circumstances and situations.

Maturity always involves knowledge of the relativistic value of the meaning of things. As this relativistic attitude increases with experience, people express their desire for an absolute core by developing faith in an activity, a movement, or a religion which they hope will compensate for the progressive disillusionment which they experience when they face the relativistic nature of things. However, there are many persons who can never master the relativistic meaning of communication, nor can they ever digest the fact that the picture of the world which they possess depends upon their own system of perception. Some of these people one encounters in daily life, others are found in mental hospitals. The condition which the psychiatrist labels "psychosis" is essentially the result of the patient's misinterpretation of messages received; and the condition which we commonly label "neurosis" is the result of unfortunate attempts of a patient to manipulate social situations with the purpose of creating a stage to convey messages to others more effectively. The messages are usually not understood by others, and the result is frustration for the patient. Then the patient is forced to develop ways of handling the frustration, which procedure further distorts the processes of communication.

These general statements about communication of patients labeled psychotic or neurotic may be illustrated in greater detail. The schizophrenic patient, for example, tends to be unaware of the fact that human relations are multi-polar phenomena; he assigns himself a role and neglects the fact that roles are determined by a mutual relationship. In the past this phenomenon was called autistic thinking; we prefer to see it as a distortion which makes a schizophrenic unaware of his impact upon others, though he maximizes the coercive aspects of the messages which others may have for him. After all, that which we call a role is simply a code which indicates in what way a message to one's self and to others is to be interpreted. This distortion of communication prevents the schizophrenic, first, from receiving messages correctly and, second, from correcting information which he already possesses. Unable to correct his incorrect information, he progressively builds a distorted model of himself and of the world. Such views result in progressive isolation, inasmuch as distorted information renders impossible appropriate interaction with others.

The psychoneurotic patient, in contrast, seems to suffer from a different type of distortion. By and large he tends to flood others with messages, in an attempt to coerce them into accepting roles they are not willing to assume. These compulsive attempts to shape situations and coerce people obviously result in unsatisfactory interaction. Neurotics, instead of correcting the messages which they transmit unsuccessfully, essentially re-peat the same message over and over in the hope that eventually it will be understood. If the term "psychosis" is reserved for people whose communication processes are primarily disrupted in the sphere of perception, the term "neurosis" refers to dif-ficulties in the area of transmission of messages to others. All neurotic patients attempt to influence the behavior of others. The hysterical personality, for example, uses demonstrable bodily signs to communicate with others, and the psychopathic personality favors actions which will please or displease the other person. The compulsive intellectual and the fanatic broad-cast their messages uninterruptedly and attempt to influence others without being concerned with the actual effects of their actions upon people; only the mature person is aware of the reciprocal effects of communicative actions and of the beneficial effects of successful human relations.

The immature person (141) is the principal bearer of psycho-somatic manifestations. Unable to interrelate themselves as ma-ture people do, these patients still use the means of communica-tion which prevailed in their early childhood. This implies that in interpersonal communication, impressions derived from the chemical and sensory end organs prevail over impressions re-ceived from the more complex distance receivers—that is, vi-sion and hearing. Significant messages, therefore, are preferably transmitted by such individuals in an intimate person-to-person contact which involves touch, pain, temperature, or vibratory, olfactory, and gustatory functions. The physical symptoms are frequently used for purposes of communication; these, so to speak, represent areas of contact which dominate human re-lations. Some skin diseases, many allergic manifestations of the respiratory tract, and some conditions afflicting the upper and lower intestinal tract and the peripheral vascular system may be mentioned as examples (135), (136), (142), (150).

Psychosomatic patients are inclined to assume that other people follow the same system of codification-evaluation that they themselves possess; for practical purposes this amounts to the assumption that they and the other person are part of one and the same physical matrix or neural network. This assumption of course held true with regard to the patients' relationship to the mother before birth, and they do not seem to have learned that in interpersonal communication, messages have to be transmitted in space and have to be repeatedly recodified. Furthermore, these immature personalities tend to weigh unduly the information which they receive from their own body by means of proprioception, to the neglect of the information received from the outside world by means of exteroception. Hence they are unable to evaluate correctly the effect of their own actions upon others, and therefore they are unable to correct their information, in regard to a constantly changing environment. Another way of stating this is to say that the delineation of the physical, psychological, and social boundaries of such patients are either incomplete or arbitrary. Because of such distortions, individuals have to place reliance upon the protective actions of others, rather than being intent upon gaining information through interaction with contemporaries.

At this moment the critical reader may raise the question of how the "organic" diseases of the body fit into the concept of communication. Without reservation it can be stated that even physiologically oriented psychiatrists, who use shock therapy and lobotomy as modes of therapy, implicitly use the concept of communication. All physicians have as their aim the improvement of the instruments of communication, and the neurologist and neurosurgeon concentrate especially on the central nervous system, which is in fact the most important organ of communication. There exists really no fundamental difference between the psychotherapist who deals with the functional aspects of the interpersonal system, the social scientist who is concerned with the larger superpersonal systems, and the physiologist who copes with the interaction of an organism with his surroundings in terms of physical and chemical events. To express this idea in more abstract terms, one can say that physiologist, psychologist, and psychiatrist alike are concerned with problems of order and disorder, entropy and the maintenance of the organism; the difference between these scientists is that the physiologist is concerned with the exchange of calories and chemical elements, and the psychiatrist and psychologist with the exchange of information (181).

These brief examples may suffice to illustrate the meaning of disturbed communication as it is observed in psychiatric patients. While it is beyond the scope of this volume to build a new psychopathology based upon criteria of communication, the reader may be reminded that in the active practice of psychotherapy, criteria of communication are used for the operational assessment of interpersonal events taking place between patient and therapist (149). From meeting to meeting, the psychiatrist assesses the state of communication which exists between himself and the patient, and in the course of time practically the whole gamut of disturbances of communication are encountered in any one patient. Granted that each patient has some more or less stereotyped disturbance, we nonetheless cannot neglect the fact that psychiatrists and other observers are struck by the change which occurs in the system of communication of these patients over a period of time. The old psychopathological diagnoses become rather meaningless in view of the flux in the means of expression which these patients use. The only thing that the psychiatrist really can rely upon is the state of communication as it is observed at a given moment, within a given context, and involving specific people. At a different date, in a different context, and with different people, the means of communication of the patient may appear in a totally different light. It seems that criteria which denote the range of disturbances of communication as well as the optimum level of functioning which a patient can reach are operationally more useful criteria than statements describing a given condition at a given moment. After all, a diagnosis always implies that a given condition is present most of the time; it introduces a typology rather than a functional appraisal of the patient's system of communication, and typologies, though useful at times, often introduce undesirable distortions. And this the therapist attempts to avoid.

The task of the modern therapist can be compared to the task of the maintenance engineer or of the trouble-shooter who repairs the great overland power lines. The therapist aims first at understanding disturbances of communication, and as a result of this, to correct defective processes of communication. This not only involves the undoing of already established patterns, but frequently necessitates the teaching of the basic elements of human communication. If circumstances and people are kind to the new-born child, the infant will enjoy, as a baby, through childhood and adolescence, the benefits of an environment where people are both aware of, and seek the pleasure of, communication. But countless thousands are born in surroundings that scorn communication and never have an opportunity to acquire the means of communication (141). Such people are potential or actual psychiatric patients. Whyte (179) states that "thought is born of failure"; we should like to add that communication is a balsam which heals the wounds acquired in the battle for life. These people who have not mastered communication have difficulty in handling frustration, and frustration itself is a deterrent to the learning of successful communication. This vicious circle the psychiatrist aims at interrupting.

It is beyond the scope of this volume to describe the operational procedures of the therapist. What we are attempting to do is to point out the close relationship between problems of biology, anthropology, and psychiatric practice. The notions which underlie psychotherapeutic practices are all expressions of the communication systems prevailing in a given culture. We have pointed out before the close relationship between value theory and communication, and it is needless to say that the notions of health and sickness, sanity and insanity, and the styling of therapeutic methods are a function of cultural values —that is, of the communication systems prevailing in a given area. Indeed, all therapeutic methods derive their media such as language and gesture, and the way they are handled, from the social matrix as a whole. Whenever the therapist is attempting to help the patient, he and the patient form an interpersonal network of communication which in turn is a part of a larger group and cultural network.

It is the task of the psychiatrist to help the patient to acquire means of communication which will help him to adjust to the group and cultural network prevailing in his surroundings. Fundamentally all people can be helped to improve their means of communication. Only the level at which patient and doctor start their work varies; some patients are very sick, some are better off, and the speed of improvement fluctuates depending upon a variety of factors. But over a period of years, and without exception, improvement can be observed if the patient has the motivation to improve and the desire to survive.

4 · COMMUNICATION AND AMERICAN VALUES: A Psychological Approach

By Jurgen Ruesch

IN DEVELOPING our thesis, we have shown so far that the verbal and non-verbal procedures of psychiatrists are designed to improve the processes of communication of their patients. The systems of communication of both psychiatrists and patients are in turn derived from the wider social matrix in which doctor and patient operate. While the conventional relationships are clearly defined in terms of the culture in which they occur, the more deviant relationships and methods of communication encountered in psychiatry are likewise embedded in the superpersonal networks of group and culture. The next three chapters, therefore, are devoted to a discussion and illustration of the more specifically American features of the social matrix and their relationship to present-day therapeutic practices.

A great many schemes (7), (9), (23), (32), (47), (49), (65), (69), (82), (86), (95), (98), (102), (112), (157), (167), (175) have been suggested for understanding the psychology of the American people, and depending upon the purpose for which an approach was designed, they have had their advantages, disadvantages, and distortions. The method which we are going to present in this chapter is characterized by the fact that we have attempted to understand some basic characteristics of human communication in America. Though the Anglo-Saxon countries have many similarities in their systems of communication, it would be a mistake to assume that the systems of evaluation are identical or even similar in all the countries where English is spoken. For example, the general rules which pertain to the interpretation of messages in the United States are not only based upon the symbols, words, and gestures used, but include such subtle things as timing and spacing of messages, the evaluation of figure-ground phenomena, the interpretation of authority, child-raising practices, and many other features.

In the scheme which we have followed, the American psychology has been described as being governed by the premises of equality, sociality, success, and change, which are thought to be interconnected by the multiple premises of puritan and pioneer morality. These four values, together with the core of moral principles, can be conceived, on the one hand, as pivotal points around which American life revolves, and on the other, as cornerstones upon which communication is based. Each of these values either may refer to goal-directed behavior or may express an intermediate implementation, instrumental to a more remote goal. Accordingly, messages exchanged regarding these activities or purposes must be interpreted in the same light. Therefore, when we as scientists make statements about value premises which prevail in the American culture, we refer on the one hand to the written or verbal comments about activities, and on the other hand to the experiences which are the result of participant action. It follows that these premises are a code for the interpretation of statements about actions and of actions themselves.

In reading the analysis of American values to be presented here, the reader will feel that the authors are biased in one way or another. Far be it from us, the authors, to deny the correctness of such a feeling. Rather, we would remind the reader that it is the essence of epistemology to view one system in the light of another. Depending upon the choice of the second system, this or that feature will by contrast appear to be exaggerated or perhaps even distorted. In the present and subsequent chapters we have chosen to look at America from a western European perspective; if we were more familiar with other cultures we might have chosen a South American or Chinese standard of comparison.

Furthermore, in discussing cultural premises and in developing generalizations about the behavior of people, everybody is able to cite, for practical purposes, examples of an antithesis which would contradict the thesis presented by the authors. However, such contradictions are to be expected. In part they are due to the fact that the data used for deriving generalizations belong to the historical past, and that in the meantime the situation has already changed; in part, they may be based on selective experiences of both author and reader; and in part they may be due to the levels of abstraction at which statements are interpreted. As a general rule, it may be stated that contradictions can usually be resolved either by interpreting a statement at a higher level of abstraction or by breaking a statement down into its more concrete components. Be that as it may, such difficulties are unavoidable, but to us as authors, it seems as if the gain of such an analysis is greater than the loss associated with a lack of understanding of such superpersonal systems. With this in mind, the following paragraphs were written.

PURITAN AND PIONEER MORALITY

The wave of Protestantism which is associated with the names of Luther, Calvin, Huss, Zwingli, and others found its way to England, where it was identified first with the Reformation and later with the Puritanism of Cromwell. The core of Puritan morality was pietism, the deprecation of carnal passion, the high valuation of self-control and will power, and the assumption of personal responsibility vis-à-vis God. The Puritan valued plain living, industriousness, thrift, cleanliness, consistency, honesty, and favored simplicity of worship and cooperation with other members of the Puritan community. All these values derived from an oppositional tendency of British Puritans, a protest—both political and religious—against the existing conditions in Europe. Broadly, the Puritans strove for simplicity and coherence; and the confusion against which they strove may well have been due to cultural heterogeneity. The ideas of the Renaissance gradually seeped through the mass of the population, creating contradictions of value and belief and abuses of action which many may have found intolerable. To escape from the anxieties of multiple choice and lack of direction, the Puritans originated certain rigidities of behavior in order to obtain a long-lost security. The systems they set up met opposition, and they left the scene in protest (172).

They arrived in America on a new continent inhabited by hostile Indians and with a rigorous climate of rugged winters and hot summers. They had to cope with hardship, and under these totally different living conditions the Puritans developed what we here call the pioneer morality. Because they were few in number their lives were valued; in order to survive, they needed rugged individuals who were well versed in the techniques of fighting nature and Indians, able to grow their own food and to clear and cultivate the earth. Adaptability to changing situations and suddenly arising emergencies was valued. There was little time for pleasure if a man wanted to survive, and hard work was his lot. The initial shortage of women, especially in frontier outposts, reinforced the rigid rules regarding behavior toward the opposite sex, which the Puritans brought with them. The first settlers were likewise faced with the necessity of setting up social relations which would favor a closely knit group because the odds against them were great and could only be overcome by superior organization. The fusion of the needs of the pioneers with those of the Puritan constituted the root of the American value system. (23), (126).

Subsequently this system was modified by the shift from an agrarian to an industrial-metropolitan economy, by the influx of non-Puritan settlers, and by all those changes which were brought about by the rise of a modern technical civilization.

Pioneer and puritan morality is the core of the American value system. The actual history is, however, not immediately relevant. For the present inquiry it is more important to note that currently, today, there exists a pride in this core of the culture. American youngsters meet a whole literature of truth and fiction romanticizing the frontier and extolling the values which it supposedly fostered. While he is absorbing these notions about the past, the young American is also receiving a barrage of other value-forming impacts from comic magazines and gangster serials, and he is being initiated by other publications into the excitements of engineering and mechanics. These other value-forming sources might seem to contradict the messages of the puritan and the pioneer, but actually the contradiction is only superficial. The virtues extolled are still the same: toughness, resourcefulness, purpose, and even purity.

Also in accord with the traditional pattern, the arbiter and censor of American morals is no single individual; instead, authority is vested in the group. Where the European child defers to his parents and a European adult defers to identifiable persons with real and sympathetic authority, the adult American defers to the collective opinion of his peers. This social organization and its reinforcement of morality is characteristic of a society of equals. Actions which violate other American value premises become acceptable when the principle of moral purpose is not violated. These tendencies are clearly reflected in the procedures which exonerate sharp practices, if they were undertaken in the name of free enterprise and rugged individualism. In the American judicial system, the municipal judges have a freedom to rule unparalleled in other countries; they really interpret the meaning of morality, and as long as the rulings do not conflict with the major premises of the American value system, their decisions will usually be upheld in higher courts.

This peculiar role which morality occupies in American life explains in part the many contradictory trends which puzzle the foreign observer (95). A foreign traveler is made aware of moral principles in situations where impulse gratifications have to be justified. He will recognize that pleasure cannot be indulged in for its own sake; this fact is epitomized by the saying that a puritan can have anything he wants as long as he doesn't enjoy it. Gratifying a personal need is permissible when justified by a socially acceptable motive. For example, recreational pleasures, vacations, sexual intercourse, eating, and all other pleasures become acceptable as long as these activities are undertaken for the purpose of promoting one's own or other people's health.

Another socially acceptable motive is the welfare of the community. In the American system, the stronger person assumes responsibility for the weaker one as long as the weakness is the result of age or circumstance. Weakness owing to lack of will power or to laziness or carnal passion is not tolerated; and the saying goes: "Never give a sucker an even break." A series of institutions take care of the less fortunate people, and everyone tries to help those who through no fault of their own become ill or lose their homes. Such help is rarely outright charity; by and large it is offered in terms of loans or other temporary relief measures. Actions which improve the social welfare or which contribute toward the general raising of standards of living are acceptable for justifying impulse gratifications. Making money, for example, even if it involves ruthless exploitation of others, can be rationalized as being necessary for supporting the family or sending the kids to school, or for some other moral purpose such as providing for the future or starting a business to create employment for others.

The regulation of impulse gratifications has found its repercussion in the American Constitution. The 18th Amendment, for example, introduced prohibition to Americans. Likewise the Mann Act was designed to curb prostitution. A similar purpose is accomplished by the Johnston Office, which, established by the movie industry, acts as a censoring or self-censoring body controlling the "morals" of the movies. It is of interest to note that American motion-picture producers, the church, and the public consider murder, violence, and brutality a perfectly moral subject for presentation in movie houses, where youngsters of all ages are admitted. In contrast, pictures which refer to sexual intercourse or which unduly expose the body are banned. Brutality and toughness are considered necessary for survival, while sensual pleasure is believed to soften the individual. A similar ideology is found in the rules governing the transportation of immoral material in the United States mails.

Inasmuch as the individual is quite aware of his impulses, Americans develop their own methods for gratifying their instinctual needs. Gratification can be indulged in, if the group behaves similarly. For example, a "regular guy" is he who as a member of a group indulges in all the vices without going overboard. Behavior that is considered immoral when committed by a single person individually is acceptable and free of external sanction when committed in the presence of others. Promiscuity, gambling, and fighting belong in this category. A similar situation is encountered in the peculiar mixture of freedom, restraint, and competition practiced by adolescents in their dating and petting activities in which there is a combination of sex play, popularity contests, and group meetings. It is beyond the scope of this volume to cite the adolescent sex practices of American teen-agers; it may, however, suffice to point out that they are characterized by incomplete unions and by perversions, which at that age are accepted as normal (65), (87). These presexual games are commonly engaged in in the presence of other couples, while privacy would really act as a deterrent. The European traveler is struck by the general exhibition of familiarity prevailing at parties and in such places as "lover's lanes," where there may be hundreds of automobiles parked with young couples engaged in exploring each other. Similarly the occasion of the annual convention of the American Legion, class reunion, or a shore leave from a ship permits its members to indulge collectively in pranks, drinking, and fighting, in a manner which would not be permitted in isolated cases.

Situational conformity is considered by Americans to be a form of group service, and submission to group opinion constitutes a moral motive. Meetings are organized so that people can obtain moral approval of their actions through active participation (103). Thousands of organizations ranging from the Parent-Teacher Association, the Y.M.C.A., the Boy Scouts, to the lodge and fraternal organizations meet with the purpose of sharing a goal which in itself becomes a moral act. The church, for example, is in America a meeting house in which people engage in group conformity rather than in an individualized religious experience. Therefore the person who dares to go his own way and does not conform either in celebrating, in everyday behavior, or in intellectual or artistic pursuits is frowned upon; if, however, he finally comes through and makes good, obtaining the public's approval, he is admired by the group and past sins are forgiven. This process is shown in

countless American films of the bad man who is finally converted
and joins the good cause.

Within the family and in small groups the woman is the
keeper of the morals for man, woman, and child. In the presence
of women, men will dress up and behave. As a matter of fact,
they strain themselves to live up to the expectations of the
female sex. Men among themselves are more likely to misbehave
and to let things ride, a fact which vividly contrasts with the
customs prevalent in western Europe, where men are considered
the carriers of morals and traditions.

In American daily life, honesty is taken for granted when it
concerns such small items as paying a nickel for a newspaper, or
leaving the milk and the mail at the door of private homes.
However, honesty is doubted when issues of power are involved.
Stealing a few cents' worth of merchandise would be such a
small crime that it is not considered worth while to risk being
caught by irate citizens or to expose oneself to the feeling of
guilt. Furthermore, some of these daily practices involve participation as citizens in the community in terms of a common
convenience for the greatest number of people. Upsetting this
system would mean elimination of milk distribution or newspapers or mail. If, however, a man is aspiring to a position of
power, as for example in politics, it is expected that he will use
his power for selfish purposes as far and as long as he can get
away with it. A man who can misuse his power and get away
with it is admired to the extent that for a long time gangsters
and racketeers became idols for youngsters, and the law-enforcing agents that could not catch them were ridiculed. The use
of aggressive and ruthless methods in the pursuit of power is
approved, but the group is expected to control any form of
corruption if it goes to excess. The control is exerted by the
press, which acts as a morality-enforcing agency. The public
suspects any man in public office; if a man were entirely honest
and interested only in the promotion of the welfare of others
he would be considered a sucker; and to be a sucker is the
worst reputation a person can acquire. Thus in America no
time and effort are spared to set up administrative procedures
to prevent fraud and other misuse of power on a large scale.

The number of forms ordinary citizens have to fill out in multiple copies, the complicated design of tax forms, and the number of things people have to swear to are unheard of in other countries. In these matters bureaucracy really flourishes.

After a man has gotten away with acquiring and using his power to the limit without being tripped, he is expected to return the yields of his success to the community. The group really engages the power-thirsty individual in a game; if people yield power to a man they want him to be selfish; only a selfish man is believed to have moral character. If he doesn't make use of his power he must be suspected of being a weakling or a fool. The group is willing to offer him an opportunity to develop his bid for power. But once his term is over the group repossesses power and wealth that were lent to the man so that it may be reinvested in another individual. Therefore, political officials are seldom elected for longer than three terms, rarely are fortunes amassed without a large amount being returned to the state in the form of either taxes or donations, and very seldom is a racketeer allowed to "do business" for more than a few years.

EQUALITY

"Fourscore and seven years ago our fathers brought forth on this continent a new nation, conceived in liberty, and dedicated to the proposition that all men are created equal." That these words have become famous demonstrates the importance of this principle in the American culture. Based upon the principle of equality, America became a melting pot of differing nationalities. Equality as practiced in daily life derived on the one hand from puritan morality and on the other from frustrating experiences of the early settlers and pioneers. Most immigrants left behind in the old country what they regarded as either an oppressive social system or an oppressive family, and once they had arrived in America they laid the foundations to prevent oppressive authority from ever arising again. By vesting functional authority in a tribunal of equals, the principle of equality was born; its specific American management thus became a solution for the immigrant's authority problem.

Today the value of equality is expressed in all those processes which result in eradication of extreme deviations and therefore promote a "regression toward the mean." Soon, however, the foreign traveler is struck by many strange contradictions: on the one hand he reads and hears about the notion of equality, while on the other hand he can observe the greatest inequality in terms of wealth, position, and power. An insider will then explain to him that in America the value of equality is interpreted as the assumption of equal opportunities rather than the product of final achievement. Once a person has become successful by exploiting the equal opportunities he has in fact become superior and unequal; though he may silently dwell upon his achieved status, he will be challenged by the popular remark, "Who do you think you are?" to remind him of his background. We thus arrive at the notion that those who achieve status, power, and wealth are presumed to have been skillful in utilizing the circumstances of equal opportunity. Once success has established a difference in prestige, those in power resent being treated as equals, while at the same time they fear their own inequality. To prevent such painful encounters very elaborate administrative setups have been organized to prevent a meeting of unequals: secretaries guard the doors of their executive bosses like watchdogs; prestige carriers isolate themselves in exclusive clubs, neighborhoods, and social gatherings; while, last but not least, the awe felt by the less successful man establishes a natural barrier to the unprepared encounters of unequals. However, if for some reason or other a meeting of unequals should occur, the external characteristics of equality are adopted by both superior and inferior. For example, during the campaign periods preceding the general elections there will appear numerous pictures showing the candidates in shirtsleeves, "hobnobbing" with farmers and industrial workers. They will call each other by their first names and behave as if they were brothers. It is as if, at the meeting of unequals, a silent conversation took place during which the superior might say, "Look here, bud, I was successful, and if you make an effort you can join our ranks," while the inferior may counter with, "I admire your success—but between you and me, we are two of a kind."

And when the persons feel that some such understanding is present they might both break into laughter to cover their uneasiness.

Americans become anxious when they meet signs of inequality. Comments made by Americans about foreign cultures indicate their disapproval of caste and openly acknowledged class systems. Whenever Americans meet people who do not readily react to group pressure they betray uneasiness; such people appear as dangerous because they cannot be checked by the usual methods. This applies particularly when the average American meets another person, American or foreign, with an outstanding record in the field of intellectual or artistic achievement. Musicians or singers are tolerated because they contribute toward entertainment and participate in group meetings, but philosophers, writers, painters, and theoreticians in the field of social or natural sciences are met with the greatest suspicion. Thinking as well as artistic expression is only tolerated along conventional lines. Original and new contributions are either flouted or totally ignored. Raids on bookstores and art shops in Boston and San Francisco regularly unearth such "shameful pornography" as reproductions of Michelangelo's frescoes in the Sistine Chapel or perhaps editions of Boccaccio's *Decameron*.

The same tendency is revealed in the political arena, where outstanding scientists, especially theoreticians, are smeared with accusations of being subversive in one or another way. Idiosyncratic thinking and feeling are in America suspect. They are resented essentially because they elude regimentation from without; and rather than acknowledge the limits of external control, the persons in power attempt to stultify individuals with special talents.

It is important to stress that in America the attempt to minimize originality and idiosyncrasy is something very different in its psychological roots from the persecution of scientists and other thinkers which has occurred in Russia and Germany. In America, it is not a matter of stamping out ideas which are subversive because they conflict with the ideology of a rigid governmental policy but rather a matter of the personal anxiety which the mere existence of the creator may provoke in some politicians or in university administrators. The thinker of new thoughts in America may be labeled as crank or crackpot, but this is probably only a convenient handle. "Any stick can be used to beat a dog"—and it is perhaps not the new ideas that Americans are afraid of so much as the fact of human differences and unpredictability which is made uncomfortably evident whenever a new idea is presented.

As long as proficiency is based upon acquired skill and training, it is acceptable. But as soon as one might have to explain achievement, rightly or wrongly, by recognizing an unusual "talent," it becomes unacceptable. These facts are clearly borne out by the behavior of American artists of the nineteen-twenties who sought refuge in Paris in order to live in an atmosphere of permissiveness; or by the conditions prevailing in the field of science today (95). American men of science probably have among their members the largest number of highly creative engineers. However, there is a lack of scientific theoreticians, and those scientific thinkers who are American citizens are, by and large, of foreign birth. The pressure to conform does not produce original personalities, and therefore this field has been left almost entirely to Europeans. Strange as it seems, if Europeans in America think or write about a new idea, it is all right; since everybody knows that they are of a different background, deviation can be tolerated. But if American science is to survive, a greater degree of freedom is needed. Inasmuch as permissiveness and tolerance of differences can be learned, a concerted effort of all those who are in responsible positions is needed if the apparent trend towards control of thought is to be reversed.

The faith that freedom and tolerance create sociable and responsible people, and the belief in the individual himself, are at stake. And soon we shall know whether the individual or the collective man, whether Western or Eastern civilization, is going to predominate.

Perception of equality sets an American at ease, knowledge of inequality creates anxiety in him. Therefore the establishment of equality for the sexes, politically, economically, and socially, has become a common and popular goal. However, in pursuing this ideal several difficulties are encountered. The first hurdle to be jumped is the reciprocal relationship between liberty and equality. In order to make people equal, their liberties have to be cut. Since they are born as unequals in terms of biological or social endowment, the forces of social cohesion must be used to make them look alike. The premise of equality impedes differentiation, and individuals cannot seek that development which, for their individual circumstances, might be best for them. They always have to look and to be like others. The American white child who at home has been implicitly taught that everybody is equal and alike is scared when he meets a Negro child for the first time, primarily because his parent is ill at ease. The premise of equality is upset, and therefore a number of precautions have to be taken to rationalize the difference; prejudice and discrimination are the end result.

In this respect America differs radically from countries such as Switzerland, for example. Both are republics; both have no caste system; both believe in liberty and equality. But Switzerland puts a higher value on liberty, which includes the notion that people are different, that they develop along idiosyncratic lines, and that such differentiation is likely to result in the greatest benefit for the individual. Switzerland thus became a country in which the greatest differences in terms of beliefs, religion, and language have been synthesized and tolerated. In America, on the other hand, equality is set before liberty (47).

This is achieved by a variety of methods. First and above all, schools and state universities assure education for all. The cult of "the average man" in newspapers, radio, and movies implicitly scorns all idiosyncratic developments. If an agency wants to elicit contributions for welfare purposes, the preservation of "the typically American home" is used as bait. Thus one invokes John and Jane Doe's "average behavior" as an example, rather than referring to the top-flight men of the nation. The same method is applied in the advertisements for home furnishings, cars, and the like. Furthermore, the "men of distinction" whose images are used in advertising are not different from other men; they are only more successful and "de luxe editions" of the average man. Care is taken to make the outward appearance of all Americans equal. The reader may be reminded of a proposed amendment to the Constitution in 1810 which sought to abolish titles of nobility or, in a totally different sphere, of the way Americans are dressed: outwardly it is almost impossible to tell from his clothes to what class an American belongs. The immigration laws are a further example of this same tendency. Legal provisions have been made for the gradual acculturation of immigrants, which provide for a five-year waiting period before full status as a citizen can be applied for; then an examination must be taken before an individual is admitted to citizenship. Such an examination provides a screening of those who cannot read, write, or understand American ideals; in other words, a check is made upon whether or not the candidates could be accepted as equals.

The premise of equality is in some way related to the management of functional authority in America. Authority resides in committees or other steering groups, and these bodies settle matters of policy. Minorities are usually represented in these leadership groups, and though they have a voice in policy-making, they will never obtain the majority vote. These committees, because of their heterogeneity, obtain public respect, and the individual citizen will defer to their opinions. Whenever an American comes in contact with a personalized authority such as a police officer or other law-enforcing agent, the attitudes which are exhibited are difficult for Europeans to comprehend. Briefly, the policeman is simultaneously a social authority and a human equal. The common denominator of these two apparently conflicting ideas is the notion of the policeman as another guy who is doing a job. Within the limits of this premise a certain amount of humor can enter and even sharp dissension can be expressed. A similar situation is encountered in offices, where the procedure labeled "sassing the boss" expresses the benevolent and friendly teasing of the man in charge because of his function as authority. As soon as a man is labeled an authority he becomes unequal, and every effort must be made to bring him back to the fold of the group and make him an equal again.

SOCIALITY

Sociality, or the tendency to form social groups, has its roots in the herd instinct of the individual. In America foremost recognition is given to this group need; as a matter of fact it has resulted in a culture of living which vividly contrasts with certain foreign civilizations, which cater to the development of object systems. At first this statement sounds paradoxical, inasmuch as America is known for its technical genius and the use of machinery in every walk of life. On second thought, however, one can understand this contradiction. Consider, for example, the way machinery is treated in America: A car is unsparingly used until it has to be replaced. Typewriters, horses, and cars are lent to neighbors and friends, and no property feelings are attached to any object. In America the object is truly subservient to life. Europeans, in contrast, have less respect for an individual's need for action and expansion, but great interest in protecting inanimate objects; the guarding of works of art, furniture, books, houses, and churches is really put ahead of the needs of the individual. These facts are clearly brought out when American families with children visit their European relatives. The American youngster, when introduced into a European home, is considered ill-mannered when he subjects the home furnishings to wear and tear and, while doing so, exhibits the boastful exuberance of youth, which is accepted with tolerance on this side of the Atlantic.

In America the process of living and of interacting with others is sought as a goal in itself. Americans treat others always as people, while Europeans in many situations will treat other people like objects or as if they did not exist. Regardless of occupation or of the job performed by an individual in America, his superiors or inferiors will always treat him as an individual. Such attitudes indicate that in the minds of the people there exists an awareness that persons have families, want to live, and need a certain environment in order to survive. In brief, in America people are always people; they never become machines or animals. The fact that life is cherished is further borne out by the many excellent provisions for saving lives in emergencies;

members of the police and fire departments, lifeguards on public beaches, rangers, members of the Coast Guard and the armed forces are trained to respect and to save lives. During World War II, the medical services of the United States Army were vastly superior to those of any other nation in terms of saving lives of wounded soldiers and rehabilitating them in civilian life. No expense is ever spared if a person is in need of rescue. In addition to these emergency measures there are in the United States all those educational institutions, public health campaigns, insurance companies, and the school health services of the medical and dental profession who do everything in their power to preserve health and promote longevity.

The treatment of persons as individuals seems to be an expression of the fact that every person is a representative and member of a group, and the group assumes the responsibility for the individual. Offense against a person is an insult against a group. The American abides by decisions of the group and recognizes it as the ultimate authority. While in the patriarchal system it is quite sufficient to abide by the rules of the chief in order to be a member of the group, in a system of equals it is necessary to please many. This is the meaning of conformance.

Conformance is encountered as a consideration in practically everyone's mind. One "can't do that," "it isn't done," and "he is impossible" are examples of comments which denote the preoccupation with conformance. "Keeping up with the Joneses" is an activity of conformance which permeates social life, the purchasing of homes, automobiles, and household appliances and induces people to join clubs, to contribute to welfare organizations, and to donate their time for worth-while causes. However, adjusting one's own actions to conform to those of others always has a competitive undertone. While the American conforms to the actions of others, he is at the same time concerned with doing things "bigger and better." Hence, in America, conformance, competition, and group membership are always found together.

In order to sustain group membership the American has to be gregarious. The value of gregariousness has its roots to some extent in the circumstances of the first settlers and pioneers, who were forced to share in order to protect themselves against a hostile environment; hence getting along in a group was essential for survival. Furthermore, gregariousness is in some ways a substitute for the extended family, which frequently is not available to the American. Either family members live far apart and spread over the continent, or part of the family has remained in Europe. In the course of time, therefore, sociability became a national feature. Today it is associated essentially with middle-class behavior, which is closely identified with the national characteristics of Americans. The value which is placed upon smooth functioning and a friendly front, low intensity and avoidance of deep involvement, as well as readiness to disengage from the existing relations and to enter new human relationships, may be termed sociability. In America this personality feature is frequently taken as one of the most important criteria in assessing adjustment.

The American becomes uneasy when he finds himself alone. To be left alone is a situation to be carefully avoided; girls accompany each other to the rest rooms or for coffee in the afternoon, and boys and girls have roommates, rarely live alone, and practice double-dating. Not only do bathroom, eating, and social habits of Americans portray this fact, but it can also be observed in the arrangement of houses, or the structure of resort places. In America houses are built close together even if the owners could well afford much larger lots; in public parks and on the beaches picnickers join one another and one group attracts the other, all avoiding isolation. The foreign traveler who with an open eye inspects the American scene is amazed at the public facilities which have been created for fostering and accommodating gregarious people. From the national parks and picnic grounds to the playgrounds in smaller communities, from the commons in New England towns to the squares of western cities, there are always facilities which enable people to meet. Grange halls and lodge buildings provide meeting places for specific groups which are set aside for social gatherings. Likewise do state and federal government provide for calendar festivals such as Thanksgiving, Fourth of July, Labor Day, Memorial Day, and the like, which provide an opportunity for family gatherings or larger group reunions. In brief, Americans always travel in a group. Lacking associates is a sign of not knowing how to win friends, of not being sociable. In America one associates with others to give the impression of popularity, and if one is popular, one makes more friends. These, of course, disperse when the barometer of popularity declines. This American concept of popularity contrasts with the concept of friendship in Europe; there the test of real friendship comes when hardships and difficult situations make associations survive.

The American form of sociability, which we have termed sociality, finds its climax in the cocktail party. Any foreign traveler is puzzled when he attends this peculiar metropolitan institution for the first time in his life. The first impression he receives is that all or most of the participants are slightly intoxicated. He then will learn that alcohol permits the American to promote his patterns of sociability. In a social situation actions which would otherwise be frowned upon become acceptable when committed under the influence of alcohol. Such behavior is characterized by patterns of increased familiarity, regardless of whether it consists of making a pass at a member of the opposite sex, or whether it is expressed in increased chumminess with a member of the same sex. To have been drunk together is a seal of friendship and insures greater popularity. Hence at the cocktail party there is a large crowd of people, all attempting to be popular, speaking a few sentences with one person and then going on to the next. Many people loathe cocktail parties, but most people eagerly attend them. It is a place where information is exchanged, popularity ratings are established, new acquaintances are made, and the general status of in-group membership is verified.

The host who gives the party usually makes a "social effort" to improve his position by breaking into new circles and by collecting more interesting people. Social effort, which is greatly appreciated in America, denotes the attempt of the individual or group of individuals to obtain votes through some sort of campaigning. This social effort not only permeates the life of society but is also found in business and politics. The political candidate combines wisdom with sociability, and the salesman shows a combination of friendly coercion with a need to remain popular. The value of such social effort is unofficially stressed and communicated in the schools and recreational system of America by all the pamphlets and books and friendly advice on how to join an association, how to become a member of a club, how to join an exclusive social clique, and how "to win friends and influence people" (38). Social effort can be tested and proved by winning the popularity rating in dating and dancing in high school, by obtaining a high Hooper rating, by being proclaimed the best-dressed woman of the year, or just by "making the papers."

In this perpetual atmosphere of campaigning in all walks of life, the foreigner is likely to misunderstand the cues of familiarity and intimacy. Superficial and stylized cues of sociability are interpreted by foreigners as deeper, personal interest. In fact, such cues are meant only as an encouragement to the stranger to participate freely at gatherings and thereby to add to the popularity of his American host. On the other hand, the foreigner's habit of not giving superficial cues of sociability is interpreted by Americans as arrogance or hostility. The American, who is extremely conscious of action cues, forgets that the European is less conscious of action; however, the European compensates for this unawareness by including in his own consideration all the style cues derived from objects, belongings, dress, and other personal expressions inherent in a situation, of which the American is usually less aware. The social meeting of European and American is on the whole a beautiful example of how the same events are interpreted in different ways because the two persons do not possess the same system of communications.

The group-oriented American is very conscious of his own status within his group, and he is much less aware of the status of his group as a whole among other groups. The reverse is true of the European. An American is usually conscious of whether his fellow-citizens look up to him or down on him, and to him it is more important to be liked than to like. This sensitive response to status appreciation is in part the result of the American system which enables a person to change his group if he wishes to do so. Such change may be termed "social mobility" (170). A person who has reached the top of his own group may join the group which is next higher in the hierarchy of prestige, and in the opposite direction, a person is also permitted to decline by lowering his standards of living. The individual who is "on the make" for a higher degree of prestige achieves his goal by joining a different set of associations, clubs, or lodges; he may move to a better neighborhood, buy himself a bigger car, or try to crash some rather exclusive social clique. Social mobility is an accepted phenomenon, and whoever succeeds in entering a new group is admired because of his social success. This fact is clearly borne out in the reports concerning assessment of candidates for office, schools, and clubs. Decisions are not only weighted in favor of the ability to get ahead. By and large it is safe to state that the social climbers possess a greater skill in social techniques and above all are well versed in the use and application of sociability (140), (145).

The American's basic need to move in a group and his concern with sociability have led to a far-reaching organization and differentiation within the group. From earliest childhood, the child is trained to become a member of a team; baseball, football, and basketball are training grounds for later industrial research and military teams, while fraternities and lodges in the recreational sphere, or town meetings and other organizations in the political sphere, provide the necessary training for teamwork. Every American knows how to behave and how to fit into the organization of a group. Adjusting to the group and engaging in teamwork brings marked advantages to the individual. The group protects its members when they get into trouble with members of other groups, or when disease or disaster strikes. The sort of reliance that an Englishman would derive from the knowledge that the judicial system and the police look out for law and order, the American citizen derives from the knowledge that the group will support him and if necessary exert pressure to protect him. Therefore, no American will shy away from expense or effort to join a team and to subordinate himself to its over-all purpose, and in return, to expect some security from the team for having "played ball."

SUCCESS

In America success is a yardstick with which the value of an individual is measured; it is the result of effort, initiative, and luck (88). We use the word "yardstick" because, in practice, the success of any individual can be gauged only by comparing it with the success of others; for this purpose external, quantifiable measures are needed. Finally, if an individual is labeled as successful by his peers it means that "everything is going his way."

In America the prevalent motivation for seeking success is found in the attempt of the individual to secure his own future against the imputed skepticism of others. At a deeper psychological level it is related to a need for approval from peers and equals and to an urge for elbowroom. Needless to say, the historical root of this national ideal of Americans is found in conditions such as the open frontiers, the unlimited possibilities, and the Industrial Revolution. In a fluid frontier society, success was the only measure by which contemporaries could gauge a man's position within his group. Therefore, success in whatever was started became the basis upon which respect and confidence from others could be secured. At the same time the notion of having been successful strengthened the self-respect of an individual, while some degree of self-confidence was necessary to initiate success. This vicious circle is best expressed by the saying, "Nothing succeeds like success."

The mushrooming growth of success has a fatally attractive and infectious effect upon others; "For unto everyone that hath shall be given, and he shall have abundance; but from him that hath not shall be taken away even that which he hath" (Matthew xxv:29). The American will gamble for the sake of success; he will play the horses and the stock market, he will participate in gold and uranium rushes, and he will invest in ventures of all sorts even at the risk of being one of many who will perish. However, if he wins, he is going to be the man who made good, demonstrating to his peers that he has left behind suppression and exploitation, that he is worthy of the attention and admiration of his contemporaries, and that he can be trusted to carry things to a successful conclusion.

The tendency to evaluate actions and things in quantitative terms is a tendency so strong among Americans that they themselves laugh about it. One might speculate that the root of quantification was found in the situation of the pioneer: Not having any information about the character or personality of a settler, none the less one urgently needed his help. Because statements out of the mouth of a stranger could not be trusted and because the various pioneers frequently came from different backgrounds, the scales necessary to evaluate a person were not uniform. To prevent misunderstanding, objective and quantifiable terms had to be used, and thus a man's position was determined by his measurable success rather than by convention and tradition. The tendency toward quantification was further promoted by the whole economic trend of the Occidental culture, the rise of commerce, and the Industrial Revolution with its emphasis upon a monetary economy. The presence of a large immigrant population and the constant change in social attitudes resulting from acculturation and social mobility produced a society in which many individuals lived in a social setting in which the major premises were fundamentally different from those of the society in which they had grown up. This diversity of premises and means of communication has the effect of guiding the individual toward the simplest possible statement, the statement in terms of quantities.

Once the tendency toward quantification was established, this tendency became self-promoting. No longer were there persons unable to find a common ground for value agreement, but instead any stranger facing another stranger could rely upon the tacit understanding that action and achievement were to be evaluated in quantitative terms. This shared premise gradually became culturally standardized, and in its most abstract form it became a system of interpretation and evaluation in the realm of communication. Needless to say, the quantitative attitude of the American acts in social intercourse as a pressure which further tends to maximize the quantifiable aspects.

There is no reason to believe that the human organism has an instinctual trend toward quantification. Indeed, what we know of mammalian background would indicate that mammals seek optima rather than maxima of the various conditions which they require. These optima are elements which are so complex that their achievement could only be measured in parameters much more abstract than any normally used in daily life. Therefore, when human beings started to exert pressure upon individuals to act in certain ways in neglect of their own instinctual needs, the possibility of the maximization of variables appeared.

The maximization of quantifiable variables makes its appearance early in childhood. American parents implicitly demand of their small children that they be heavier, bigger, stronger, and smarter than other babies. Love is given conditionally, and only if the baby talks and walks earlier and is "cuter" than other babies will he obtain more love than those who are second or last in the quest for success. The American child has the problem of stating achievement in terms which shall be so demonstrable and so convincing that parents must assent to his demands. The obvious and natural solution to this problem is for the child to take over quantitative cues from the parents. As he grows older he will boast of his marks at school and of how little effort he has put into achieving them; of how many times he has swum the length of the pool, and of how much money he has earned from selling newspapers.

The parent or leader faces a similar problem, inasmuch as he has to find value propositions which will evoke agreement in a number of persons whose value systems he presumes to be different from his own. If, for example, a public speaker desires a certain policy to be accepted, he has the task of making others desire this policy also, though their reasons may be different ones. In such a situation the bare agreement on policy has to be shared and all the ideas which might obscure the issue must be shorn off. This means that the suggested policy must be torn away from the complex matrix of each individual's idiosyncratic beliefs and expectations. The result may be a slogan, or it may be a list of separate objectives, or it may be a simple quantitative statement to which all can agree. Thus out of the process of reducing a spectrum of opinions to a single statement emerges the tendency to quantify actions, which affects the whole of American life.

One of the universal indexes of an individual's success is his income, property, or other manifestations of wealth. Thus Americans talk about a "fifteen-hundred-dollar fur coat" or "a forty-thousand-dollar home" rather than describe what sort of fur coat or home they are talking about. Likewise the prestige of a person increases with salary, and Americans talk about "a twenty-thousand-dollar-a-year job." If an individual achieves success in administration or engineering, and his responsibilities are rewarded by a good, but not a top, salary, it is common to translate the prestige gained into monetary terms by imagining the sort of financial position which he could claim. He is, however, given credit for not claiming this position if he so chooses. A Secretary of State, for example, is respected not so much because he is a Secretary of State but because, if he should resign his job, he could claim the chairmanship of a board or the position of the president of an industrial or trust company at many times the salary he receives in government service.

The actual achievement is not the only aspect of success which Americans value. As long as anyone strives for success, as long as he makes an effort, he is a regular guy. This striving has to be smooth, casual, and shrewd, and the effort must not show. The intention to seek success is a socially acceptable motivation, while instinct gratification as such is rejected. It is perfectly permissible, for example, for an American to say that he has joined a lodge system, such as the Rotary, Lions, Masons, Moose, or Elks, or a church group, for the sake of insuring future success. Likewise a boy is sent to college not so much for the sake of learning as for an opportunity to make contacts with other boys of more prominent families, contacts which are considered a stepping stone to success. While a man who is successful becomes the object of competition and envy, the man who is starting out and who tries hard is the person to whom the already successful persons give a chance and lend a hand. "There's no harm in trying" is a slogan which denotes the appreciation of effort in America.

Making good is a relative achievement; and, as the saying goes, one should not "play ball in the wrong league." This definition of success clearly implies that success is to be judged

by a person's position vis-à-vis his peers, and not vis-à-vis those
people who belong to another group or social class. As soon as
success has made a person distinctly different from his peers, he
has to join another league in order to continue competition with
equals. This traditional rule is clearly exemplified in the management of baseball leagues, the type of neighborhood people choose
to reside in, or the type of clubs they join. It is obvious that success is infectious, and that when it makes its appearance everyone
is ready to climb on the bandwagon. This effect seems to be a
human characteristic, however, rather than a uniquely American trait.

The end justifies the means, and success exonerates ruthless
and sharp practices. If an opportunity looms, a challenge is
automatically felt, even though responding to this challenge
might bring one into conflict with the law; but if a person is
caught cutting corners, he is considered a failure. The emphasis,
therefore, is not upon what he does but on whether others
permit him to get away with it. Rarely is an American racketeer
charged with the crime he has committed (162). Usually he is
caught not for running brothels or for smuggling narcotics or
liquor, but for income tax evasion: he is arrested for cutting a
corner but not necessarily for his major crime.

The fact that success is a goal in itself and that achievement
is more important than the methods used to obtain it is made
possible through a class society which permits vertical mobility
(170), where mastery is frequently only incidental to success.
In contrast, a caste society with its limitations of success and
social mobility promotes mastery and virtuosity as an end in
itself (158), (166). The result of this tendency can be substantiated by the fact that almost all artisans and skilled workers in
America are of immediate European descent and that American
trained workers will strive for mastery only to the point where
success is secured. American houses, for example, are built to
last only a generation, and the building of houses, both in structure and in aesthetic appearance, is determined by the needs
of the moment. To build a house which would last for hundreds
of years would in America be considered a folly. In Europe a
high degree of perfection in philosophy, art, and handicrafts is

found because the rigid class structure does not permit social mobility; instead mastery of a skill is one of the achievements from which the individual gains satisfaction. In America the acquisition of a skill is a means of securing success, and success is thought to be of the essence in the pursuit of happiness.

The American people have a rich mythology about people who have made good; the myths of Ford, Rockefeller, and Carnegie idealize free enterprise and the poor man's chance to grow rich and powerful. However, this admiration of success is combined with a condemnation of the sharp practices of the robber barons. The public, however, is willing to close an eye to questionable procedures if the behavior of a successful man is later mitigated by good works, charitable contributions, establishment of foundations and other public institutions. In contrast to the admiration shown for these business personalities the respect for a Washington, a Jefferson, or a Lincoln shows unrestricted admiration for their success and their restraint in the use of power. This is not the adoration of free enterprise or of the go-getter, but is rather an expression of admiration for rugged individualism. A similar attitude is exemplified in the slogan "from log cabin to White House," and it is supposed that those persons who gain fame and prestige through political and administrative skills earn their reputation by a wise use of power. Not only the acquisition of power but also its wise administration is a factor in earning the label of success in America. Finally we may mention the heroes like Lee, "Stonewall" Jackson, Teddy Roosevelt, and Patton, whose success was due to their ruggedness in military campaigns.

Business executives, governors of states, and presidents are entrusted with great responsibilities, and unusual powers are delegated to them. Success means the achievement of positions of responsibility and the use of power. Power need not be used exclusively for the good of the people. A governor who may be a good and efficient administrator may still be considered a sucker if he does not know how to obtain votes from various political machines or how to make compromises in order to keep himself in office. Since personal acquisition of wealth and power is a publicly acknowledged motive for men in high positions, a great many safety factors have had to be devised to curb those who would go too far on the road of self-glorification and self-interest. Provisions for limiting the power of the corporation president, the government executive, or the legislator indicate that a successful man is compared by the American public to a circus juggler who simultaneously keeps several objects in the air without failing. The achievement of success thus means that a man has not only tasted but also exposed himself to danger, and has learned how to cope with it.

American public life provides individuals with the symbols and props of success. These can be used to exhibit success in order to make an impression, which technique may eventually assure further success; or they may be used to simulate a not yet existing success and thus provide a foundation for later success. It is customary, for example, to establish big offices, to drive large automobiles, to throw large parties, to act and talk as though one were wealthy, in order to impress others, even if money has to be borrowed to achieve this effect. People who engage in such actions hope that other persons will climb on the bandwagon because they are lured by the props of success; for if they do so, real success is likely to be around the corner.

CHANGE

The value of change is identified with social and material progress. Change is always for the better, and in the mind of Americans the good which has been achieved is thought to be almost irreversible. In contrast, the change which Europeans expect is always for the worse; but paradoxical as it sounds, the European notion of change, if it is accepted, has the quality of reversibility. In America one never retraces one's steps, and change, therefore, has the quality of being irreversible.

Life in America is not viewed as being static but is conceived as being in the process of continuous change. Nothing is ever settled, and change is a matter of course. In Europe that which may be viewed as inconsistency or lack of stability may in America be interpreted as adaptability and strength of character. One frequently finds people boasting about the number of occupations and jobs they have held in various fields to emphasize their adaptability to change and their eagerness to encompass the new. Likewise the ups and downs in business success may be romanticized to demonstrate the resiliency to change. A man, for example, may openly acknowledge the fact that he, at one time, went bankrupt, if in later years he can demonstrate that he again achieved success.

In America the readiness to accept and to promote change is revealed in many business procedures. The planning of organizations, construction, and development is undertaken with pleasure; previously erected structures are scrapped without regret, and consideration is given to the need for periodical renewal, inasmuch as obsolescence is feared. The preference for something new, rather than mending the old, is exemplified in the popular practice of trading in a one- or two-year-old car as soon as a more recent model is available; on a governmental scale the sale of war surplus materials documents the same trend.

The tendency to start new ventures rather than to stick to old ones requires special techniques, and the methods which are used to get a new venture going have been compared to pump priming. In order to get things going the American will not shy away from initial expenditure of money and effort, even if lack of success should mean temporary financial ruin. The basic idea which underlies these initial efforts is to increase the circulation and the turnover of money and merchandise. Once the wheel has started to turn and the inertia has been overcome, the American expects that all is going to turn out for the best. The use of money to initiate enterprises has been termed "venture capital," and much has been written to the effect that the pioneer spirit among businessmen is disappearing because legislation and high taxes have curbed all initiative.

The economic manipulation of American markets is quite different from procedures customary in Europe; first, products are advertised so that the public is prepared and alerted to receive the forthcoming products; thus a market is created by creating a shift in fashion trends, and the public's readiness to accept this change is generally great enough so that the goods are successfully sold. Advertisements such as "A change of laxative would be good for you" count on the public's readiness to accept change; and frequently enough this expectation is justified.

Social progress is, in American eyes, at least as important as material change. First of all there is a belief in the ability to change people; this attitude resulted in a rapid development of social science, social welfare, and other programs which are devoted to the study of social engineering. *How to Make Good* and *How to Win Friends and Influence People* (38) are titles of books which document this belief in social engineering, while associationism and social mobility are practices subservient to the notion of social change (170). Social mobility and acculturation are ways of behavior which are highly rewarded; social success is proof of the adaptability of people who undertake the burden of improving themselves, and therefore they become a living monument of "the American way of life": "from rags to riches."

To this concept of change and adaptation, psychiatry owes its present popularity. The fact that people can be changed, that the techniques to achieve such an end can be learned, fascinates American thinking. And much that was proclaimed in the past to be unalterable behavior, determined by heredity and constitution, now becomes accessible to change because of this refreshing attitude of American psychiatrists. While the belief in education and rehabilitation opens a new vista for many unfortunate and sick people, the notion of change creates at the same time insurmountable problems. There exists, for example, the American tradition that children should emphasize the difference between themselves and their parents, rather than adhere to the similarities. In compliance with this premise they tend to break away from home early, to ridicule the traditions of the elders, and to adhere to patterns which contrast with those of the parents. As a result, young people become isolated from their families at a time when maturation has not progressed to the stage where acceptance of great responsibilities becomes a matter of course (127).

Assumption of responsibilities at an early age deprives the young adult of the leisurely atmosphere which is necessary for successful social learning. From early childhood the American youngster is trained to push, to exert himself, and to work to the limit of his resources. He is expected to explore new grounds, to seize opportunities, and therefore to abandon the old for the new. In such an atmosphere of constant change, mastery of skills and techniques, the acquisition of information, and the clarification of the position of the self vis-à-vis the world become extremely difficult. The problems and personality disturbances which result from such hasty development are dumped into the lap of the psychiatrist, who in the course of his professional activities is constantly in contact with borderline people who do not know where they belong.

The American citizen views the present as better than the past and therefore believes that any future will be better than the present. The unknown element which is associated with the future invokes anxiety. Though this uneasiness is handled by effort and optimism, the belief in the future is vulnerable in periods of depression. Economic cycles seem to be accompanied by psychological cycles; in periods of prosperity the American believes in the future and in the betterment of mankind, and in times of depression he is shaken in his foundations and believes that the misery is going to last forever; both attitudes in turn have their repercussion in the economic sphere. Practices such as taking out life insurance and retirement programs, which emphasize the possibility of change in the future, or, in another sphere, the care for children by schools, agencies, and the private citizen, express great concern with the future. Almost every American, for example, feels concerned with the welfare of the future generation. The belief in the future, which characterizes all walks of American life, therefore results in the structuring of the parent-child relationship, which puts children first and parents second.

Americans are engineers, and therefore they have respect for science and rational procedures which permit them to develop their material culture (32). An engineer is in general interested in the question of "how," as it applies to the manipulation and alteration of the human environment. Such an attitude is clearly revealed by the development of American applied science, as seen in medicine and in mechanical, electrical, and chemical engineering. Investigation of nature as it is has much less fascination for the American than the exploration of what can be changed in nature. Therefore, applied science triumphs over basic science (95) and the arts, and action predominates over thought and feeling (109). The notion of engineering is carried into the field of human problems, and the American has the strange belief that social issues can be solved by the progress of material culture. Remarks about "new additions" to family or staff denote the materialistic treatment of social action and interpersonal relations. Inasmuch as inner experience is a less fruitful field for manipulation and engineering than the environment, Americans tend to externalize their inner experience. Externalism or the quantification of internal events by projecting these upon external objects or events characterizes the American personality. The American is geared to cope with change, to revere the gadget, to quantify, and to use action as the principal means of expression. The philosophy of behaviorism was thus a characteristic expression of American culture (171).

PSYCHIATRY WITHIN THE AMERICAN VALUE SYSTEM

On previous pages we have given a brief description of some of the values prevailing in America. Let us now consider how the American psychiatrist operates within such a value system and how he proceeds to help his patients in their adjustment to the prevailing system of communication.

The methods of psychotherapy were developed primarily in the private offices of psychiatrists and psychoanalysts who dealt with ambulatory patients. Therefore psychotherapists seem to be more effective in coping with minor problems of adjustment than with the major psychoses. In dealing with problems of adjustment, it seems fair to say that the therapist is essentially concerned with problems encompassing the patient's identity. "Identity" used in this sense refers to the questions of "Who am I?" "Where do I belong?" "What is my function?" "How can I cope with the problems that daily life presents me with?" In more technical terms one might say that problems of identity involve the clarification of roles and the specification of approaches which are suitable to implement the responsibilities assumed in a social situation. Whatever the technical terms may be which various schools (31), (62) use to denote these processes, they all deal with the clarification of functions of one individual vis-à-vis himself and others (123), (149), (159). The definition of identity, therefore, is not independent of the social matrix in which a person operates. On the contrary, the ways in which a person can relate himself to others are usually defined by the culture in which a person lives. Circumstances may be favorable or unfavorable in transmitting to an individual this knowledge of social practices, roles, and techniques which are necessary in coping with others; and as a result of continued contact with others the internal personality structure of an individual is gradually shaped (53).

Let us now consider the specifically American values which govern the establishment of what we shall call personality. In addition to the unique and purely idiosyncratic events which may influence a person's attitude, there exist certain cultural stereotypes. Americans, for example, see in the woman the keeper of morals for men, women, and children; basically a woman is considered to be equal to man in every respect; she willingly fulfills the role of being a vehicle in exhibiting the man's signs of success. On the other hand, the woman expects the man to be successful in terms of insuring an income with purchasing power, and he willingly exhibits his ability to earn, to please the exhibitionism of the woman. By and large, the woman has a stabilizing effect on the man, and slows him down in daring enterprises. In each other's presence men and women act in a more conventional manner, they tend to communicate in more formal terms, they remind each other of mutual obligations, and their interaction follows the stereotypes laid down by the principles of American morality. Men with men and women with women often have more fun and are freer than in mixed society, and advice on how to promote a business deal or how to get a man flows more freely in an exclusively male or female social group.

Madariaga (109) once characterized the English as people of action, the French as people of thought, and the Spaniards as people of passion. In such a scheme, the Americans would have to be classified as being the foremost people of action. Inasmuch as the American's awareness of role and status is closely connected with what he does for a living, an idle American is a man without an identity. Depending upon his activity, his identity changes, and the European traveler is often befuddled when he applies Latin standards to the understanding of the American. Over there, it matters what a person thinks and feels; here in America, it matters what a person does. There, identity is stabilized and independent of action; here, it changes with the activity.

Questions of identity occupy, of course, a central position in American psychotherapy. The self-respect of an American is by and large related to proper social functioning, getting along in a group, and doing things with others. Social considerations therefore play a big role in individual therapy. However, here is where therapeutic methods begin to differ from similar methods employed in Europe. It is well to remember that though the majority of psychotherapeutic schools originated in Europe, their practices and theories cannot be applied to the American scene without some modification. One of the reasons can be found in pronounced patriarchal systems prevailing in Europe which in America are supplanted by a system of equality or even by a matriarchal structure of the family. Most psychiatric schemes imported from Europe were geared to such patriarchal organization; and before applying any theories developed in Europe one has to understand that while the European family is organized like a pyramid, the American family seems to be more trapezoid in structure. Furthermore the European division of function between the two sexes is in America frequently blurred; the relative interchangeability of the parental and social functions of the two sexes is accompanied by a less clear-cut division of labor within the family. The parents act much more as checks and balances upon each other and constitute a sort of authority by combining their efforts. The child in turn is free to correct either parent, and as a result tends to identify with the vague and fluctuating climate of opinion of the family, which is the result of interaction of all of its members, rather than with any particular individual. In America, identification usually does not occur with a single person, but rather with a whole group, and is always related to action rather than to thought. It is remarkable to see how Freud's theory of identification was based upon the European family structure and how in its application to American conditions the theory had to be translated into terms which would conform to the social scene prevailing over here (see Chapter 6).

In practice the adaptation of abstract theoretical schemes to the values governing a particular social problem is automatically followed by practically every psychiatrist.

Whenever a patient seeks the help of a psychiatrist, he sooner or later reports difficulties in accepting some of the values which prevail in daily life. This conflict with cultural premises is, of course, not stated in these terms but is likely to be described in words which denote the patient's awareness of failure (140), (143). By and large psychiatrists have a permissive understanding; in the course of interviews with more than fifty psychiatrists who had derived their training from a variety of schools in different localities, the authors found that only a very few therapists, who were primarily physiologically oriented, assumed an attitude of disapproval and condemnation of what might be termed a violation of cultural premises. But regardless of whether a permissive or a condemnatory attitude prevailed, not one single psychiatrist could refrain from commenting implicitly or explicitly about the cultural premises with which he came in contact. Only in the attitudes toward these cultural premises did the therapists vary.

As a rule the permissive therapist does not press the patient for change and improvement; the patient's digression from puritan morality is overlooked, his lack of success accepted, his inequality taken for granted, and his unsociable isolation understood. The majority of therapists thus accept the fact that the patient violates or strives against the prevailing cultural premises, while only the minority condemn and thus establish themselves as arbiter between patient and society.

The permissive psychiatrist and his actions are on the whole a surprising experience for the patient. The latter is used to the fact that people in his surroundings are intent on reinforcing the prevailing cultural trends. Permission to move in a direction which differs or is radically opposed to the prevailing cultural values gives the patient confidence in the therapist, who is then identified as a kind, understanding parent. This temporary permission to move in a direction different from that prescribed by the culture enables the patient to rediscover the usefulness of those social premises by which he lives, not as something which is forced upon him, but as something which is desirable and fascinating. The method used in bringing the individual back into the fold of the culture which he rejects is to allow him to remain temporarily free from the pressure of other people and the group. The overt move away from the accepted cultural premise, either through hospitalization or in the course of ambulatory interviews, generates a covert longing for the things which the patient has opposed for so long. Ultimately, the desire to belong becomes so strong that the patient accepts the cultural premises and treats them as though they were his own discovery. It is at this point that they cease to exert a pressure. They are no longer felt as alien elements; instead they become part of the personality structure of the patient.

This permissive attitude of the psychiatrist vis-à-vis his patients under treatment can lead to misinterpretations when the method used—that is, the temporary permissiveness—is mistaken for the ultimate goal. The confusion between temporary methods of treatment and ultimate goal has given rise to a number of misunderstandings. For those who are unfamiliar with the procedures of psychiatrists it might suffice to say that the therapist acts very much like a benevolent parent who permits his children to make minor mistakes, to engage in pranks and youthful violations of codes of ethics, so that they may learn and understand the meaning and usefulness of that which the adult stands for. Unless such mistakes are made by both children and patients, they will not learn to distinguish between socially acceptable and unacceptable behavior. If actual reality testing is a necessity for the management of the present, the potential ability to test reality is the criterion of maturity.

The authoritarian therapist (24) proceeds quite differently from the permissive therapist. Conceiving himself as a representative of society, he essentially performs a function of education and indoctrination. As long as the patient improves—that is, as long as the patient progressively conforms to the psychiatrist's demands and therefore more and more conforms to that which is acceptable and normal—the psychiatrist remains tolerant. If, however, the patient should dare to move in a direction opposite to what might be thought of as normal, the psychiatrist will resort to sanctions. The leverage which the psychiatrist can exert might consist of withdrawal of week-end leaves for the hospitalized patient, or the transfer to a more closely observed ward with greater restrictions; the psychiatrist who treats ambulatory patients exerts a similar pressure by giving or withdrawing his personal approval, for which the patient longs. In other words, the authoritarian psychiatrist remains permissive and tolerant as long as the patient accepts the therapist's views and adjusts accordingly. The authoritarian psychiatrist is less interested in the solution of conflicts and tends instead to manipulate the situation in such a manner that the patient accepts the prevailing notions of normality. As long as outward behavior is normal, the patient is considered to be well adjusted, and internal conflict is thought of as the private responsibility of the patient.

The American term "adjustment" is unique, inasmuch as it cannot be translated into any other language. "To adjust" means to accept the existing values and to accept that which is viewed as unalterable reality. Adjustment therefore means blending into the group without showing any signs of deviation. Adjustment means a state of mental health, which condition becomes synonymous with the American concept of living, to strive, morally, equally, socially, successfully, for a better future. The American concept of readjustment, then, is a product of compromise between authoritarian and permissive practices of rehabilitation. Permissiveness is used for facilitating experimentation with reality, while authoritarian attitudes serve the purpose of providing the patient with a behavioral model which can be imitated.

In the implementation of the concept of adjustment American psychology, psychiatry, and psychoanalysis have developed a well-rounded "ego psychology" (8), (53). What a person does in terms of actions always has an impact on the environment and an effect on other people, and as soon as therapy and rehabilitation are concerned with action they must also in some ways be concerned with social concepts of normality, and rules pertaining to the regulation of social situations. The European counterpart of "ego psychology" can be seen in "superego" and "id" psychology, which more or less considers only intrapersonal events. In Europe a person's intrapersonal processes are considered to be of interest to the bearer only, and repercussions of inner experiences upon surroundings are minimized. Inasmuch as the European psychiatrist acts only in the name of himself and deals primarily with matters that are in some ways unique, he is individualistic and authoritarian. The American therapist acts not only in his own name but also as a representative of society, which wishes to take the patient back into the fold of the group. In this capacity he is more permissive than his European colleagues and actually wields greater authority. The difference between the American and the European therapist may be expressed by saying that the American therapist tends to be authoritative while his European colleague tends to be authoritarian (161).

Authoritative, functional authority is the product of a society of equals, and permissiveness is a product of the American premise of change. The American public, which is trained to accept and believe in feats of social engineering and manipulation of the environment, hopes that those who suffer from pathology can be made over. The premises of change and success with the belief in unlimited possibilities foster the idea of social engineering. During the war, for example, successful steps were taken to select men for all kinds of purposes. In contrast to the European, who believes in natural development and evolution, the American administrator feels a necessity to hand-pick men for a variety of purposes, and he prides himself on being able to do so. Pilots (144), medical students, politicians, and persons for administrative positions are usually hand-picked by those already in office, who believe that a man's success at forty is predetermined at the age of twenty. Determinism, however, applies in America only to success. If a person is a failure at the age of twenty there may still be hope for him to become a success at forty. This apparent inconsistency in deterministic attitudes is really an expression of the premises of success and equality. Americans believe that anybody can be a success if given the opportunity; hand-picking young men, then, means only providing them with opportunities, and those who have shown ability in the exploitation of opportunities are preferred. Those who fail to adjust in life are thought to have lacked opportunities, and in such cases psychiatry is supposed to compensate for these unfortunate circumstances.

There is an unfaltering belief in the possibilities of the individual, who is thought to be curbed by an unfavorable environment only. To improve and remedy social difficulties, so the American thinks, one has only to perfect the material culture, raise the standards of living, and give the people opportunities. However, such optimistic attitudes do not take into account the differences which exist between people. After the elementary needs for food, shelter, and clothing have been satisfied, people can be divided into several groups. Some do react to external factors, but thinking of the isolated schizophrenic patient, for example, we know that other people can lead a withdrawn life. But regardless of whether people emphasize the material culture or not, optimism fulfills a social purpose. Because of optimism American psychiatrists are much more active in the field of mental health, and through action a better understanding is gained. In contrast, psychiatrists in continental Europe, who in their skepticism become rather paralyzed, can be likened to botanists or naturalists; they are true students of psychopathology without attempting to manipulate the conditions which bring about psychopathology.

The puritanical roots of American morality which favor denial of instinctual gratification by promoting reaction formation instead, can be linked to the proverbial toughness of the American in business matters and his inhibition in the fields of artistic expression. The pioneer mentality with its premises of opportunism, self-assertion, and gambling for success develops personalities fascinated with action (7), (49), (69). The combination of puritan with pioneer psychology seems to have created human beings who are less sensitive to sensory and aesthetic pleasures and who prefer work and action to meditation. The psychiatric patient, then, is he who meditates, who does not indulge in instinctual gratifications, and who has difficulties with action; or conversely, he who has no fantasy life engages in impulse gratification and visualizes only short-term goals. In both cases adjustment breaks down because the minimal conditions for successful social learning are not fulfilled.

The cultural matrix, which earmarks the patient as a deviant, also determines the methods of treatment which are intended to bring the patient back into the fold of society. For example, we have mentioned above that Americans believe that success is a function of opportunity. One of the well-known texts on therapy with children states the same principle in the following words: "The patient is helped to help himself" (6). The American psychiatrist is thus considered an agent who provides those conditions which enable the patient to help himself. Such a definition of the function of the psychiatrist is vehemently protested by Europeans, who believe that the therapist's task is to make the patient understand his inner conflicts.

Inasmuch as the aim of rehabilitation implies that the patient be enabled to live in fair agreement with his surroundings, some difficulties may arise when the methods of rehabilitation appear to be in contradiction with the prevailing cultural principles. The American patient, for example, frequently has difficulty with free association; from daily life he is ill prepared to recognize the significance of all the talk that takes place in a therapeutic session. Very often, as a matter of fact, the therapist first has to overcome the feelings of guilt and shame of the patient when the latter relates facts about the past and verbalizes feelings and thoughts in the presence of the psychiatrist. Accustomed to expressing his feelings and thoughts in terms of activities rather than in terms of words, the patient feels that the methods of the psychiatrist are somehow strange. This tendency influences therapeutic procedures, and the technical term "acting out" refers to the fact that patients frequently demonstrate their conflicts to the psychiatrist by re-enacting them in real life. Instead of verbalizing his feelings of being rejected, for example, a patient may initiate relations with people who, after some coaxing, are willing to comply and to reject the patient. Only after dozens of such experiences does it dawn upon the patient that he himself creates the stage for such humiliation. "Acting out," therefore, is a beautiful example of a behavior pattern which is the result of misinterpretation on the part of the patient in overconformance with cultural premises. The reader will immediately recognize that as soon as the patient is willing to meditate about his conflicts and express them in therapy in terms of words, he is ready to give up some of his manipulating tendencies. Though on the surface it looks as if the patient had moved away from the cultural premises by talking about feelings and thoughts, he is in reality finally adjusting to the surroundings in which he lives.

Another example illustrating the beneficial effect of abandoning an all too rigid interpretation of the cultural values concerns the premise of success. The urge to explore the apparently unlimited possibilities and to seek success induces many patients to reach out far beyond their means, both economically and psychologically. Few people manage to adjust under the impact of a feeling of insufficiency, and those who in the end are not quite a success and have not made the grade permanently carry a chip on their shoulder (98). In a large number of American patients, we find that high ideals related in one way or another to success interfere with the acceptance of reality. The patient, so to speak, is constantly on the run, he never has time to learn anything really well, to digest an experience he has had, or to let things settle; he must push and hurry on, driven by his ideals to seek further success—and this striving is eventually responsible for his failure. If the psychiatrist, who is used to seeing patients whose lack of success has become a source of major frustration, succeeds in making the patient aware of the fact that his success fantasies prevent him from really achieving success, the patient is likely to be able to adjust.

After these brief illustrations of the influence of cultural premises upon the interaction between patient and psychiatrist we now may restate our basic concept of the therapeutic process. He who is a patient is by definition in conflict with some of the cultural premises which prevail in his immediate environment. Therapy provides, first and above all, an opportunity for the patient to express this conflict; secondly, therapy provides the patient with a person, the therapist, who may understand these difficulties; thirdly, a correction of the views of the patient can occur through interaction with the therapist, with the result that the patient's beliefs and his views of the cultural premises may change.

The therapist's ability to understand and to correct are obviously dependent upon a grasp of the cultural premises which form the matrix of his therapeutic activities (59). If he himself has a need to conform rigidly to those premises, he will be unable to help the patient, because then he will act as the person whom we previously described as an authoritarian psychiatrist. If, however, he is aware of the cultural premises in which he operates and if he has no particular need to conform rigidly to these, he will be able to tolerate permissively the deviations of the patient. The patient, moving temporarily against the prevailing cultural premises, is enabled to become more flexible in his conformance or non-conformance, and thus lay the foundations for a better adjustment.

In this chapter a concrete and psychological approach to the American culture has been conveyed to the reader, in the hope that the content, explicitly or implicitly, will contain some of the rules which are necessary for understanding and interpreting messages in the American system of communication. In the next chapter an attempt will be made to express the same in more abstract terms. The language of the scientific philosopher will be combined with the notions of the psychiatrist in an understanding of the integrative processes in America of both individual and group.

5 · AMERICAN PERSPECTIVES: An Integrative Approach

By Jurgen Ruesch

WALKING THROUGH the streets of a strange city, the sensitive traveler receives an impression of the prevailing atmosphere. He may not talk to anyone in particular, he may not be interested in the beauty of the shops, in the efficiency of the transportation system, or in the excellence of the restaurants, yet by just sitting, or walking, or looking at buildings, and in some impersonal way by watching the people in the streets, he begins to understand. After a little while he may engage in a conversation with the sales clerks in the stores, with the employees in his place of lodging, or with casually met acquaintances. As he continues to study he may gather information of a more concrete nature, he will begin to read about the country he is visiting, he will consult tourist guides or history books, until he begins to comprehend what it is all about.

We have made an attempt to conceptualize this sort of understanding. The specific symbols used in expressing these observations are obviously of an abstract nature; for example, they are not related to the excellence of the coffee brewed in the breakfast shop, nor do they have to do exclusively with the beauty of the women, or with the stylistic purity of the cathedrals. Instead, events perceived in strange surroundings are analyzed by the human observer in such ways that a comparison of the most divergent impressions becomes possible.

SPACE PERSPECTIVES

Space perspectives are usually the first conscious and unconscious concern of tourists. Arriving in a strange place by sea, air, rail, or road, the sightseer finds his attention involuntarily attracted by landscapes and buildings. Soon his gaze will follow the lines of the buildings, trees, mountains, and valleys. After some sight-seeing the traveler will have gained an intuitive understanding of the natives' appreciation of space. The American cities, with their relatively narrow streets and tall skyscrapers, undoubtedly reveal a vertical orientation of the architects who designed them. As the traveler gets acquainted with the people of the country, he will discover that buildings and towers are not the only documents revealing the emphasis on height. The American population also admires tall people, and this tendency has found its monument in the Paul Bunyan legends. After the traveler has decided that the vertical orientation dominates the plan of eastern cities, he becomes utterly confused when traveling west. There he encounters wide open spaces and rambling ranch houses which emphasize the horizontal perspective. After some thinking about these apparent contradictions, he comes to the conclusion that Americans are in need of expansion, be it vertical or horizontal, and that depending upon the space available, the orientation will go in either of the two directions, or both. In America, things are big.

Side by side with all this bigness in the works of nature we find bigness in the man-made objects for daily use. Cars, refrigerators, radios, desks, and other objects are frequently oversized. But when it comes to the utilization of space in homes, office buildings, and public institutions, we suddenly find thrift and an economic utilization of space. The European misses large open places in front of buildings, and squares in the center of town, and he is struck by the smallness of rooms in private homes and the absence of entrance halls. This apparent conflict between a tendency towards bigness and the principle of economy is one of the puzzling features of American life.

On gaining a preliminary orientation along vertical and horizontal coordinates and on understanding the compromise in the treatment of space, the traveler is struck by the absence of a perspective in depth. In the landscaping the European misses the contrast between foreground and background, and he is puzzled by the sudden transitions of themes; as he approaches a building from the street, often nothing but a door separates the living room from the sidewalk, and the absence of spacious entrance halls is apparent in many of the commercial structures in downtown areas. The façade of modern buildings is usually not structured in depth; on the contrary, the frontages are flat and houses close to the street. Suddenly the traveler is reminded of the fact that this abruptness and absence of transition can likewise be observed in the behavior of the people. A man may change his job or move to another part of the country without notice, or he may without any warning leave the dinner table after a lengthy conversation by just uttering three words—"Please excuse me."

While the traveler reflects upon the matter of perspectives he makes the strange observation that in spite of the many places that serve excellent food, few if any permit a view of the landscape. If views exist, they are sweeping and rarely framed by foreground, background, or lateral lines. He discovers that views exist from lookouts that have to be climbed by foot, escalators, or elevators, but that these same views are rarely incorporated in daily life in the living or dining rooms of the people. On the contrary, the buildings are frequently arranged in such a manner that people look upon enclosed spaces. Since in America, nature is frequently hostile to people, views seem to be threatening, and only immediate, man-made surroundings appear to be comforting and friendly. Thus American houses have patios, lawns, and terraces rather than views. This tendency contrasts with the situation in Europe, where throughout the centuries the soil has been worked over and over until the views which one can have through windows always embrace friendly and man-tamed nature.

TIME PERSPECTIVES

Upon closer contact with the American scene and its inhabitants it becomes clear that the coutry's orientation leans towards the future. First of all, there is a future, and the future is going to be better than the present; therefore it is eagerly anticipated and the people are full of infinite immediacies. The attitude towards the past, the present, and the future seems to be related to the ability to manipulate, construct, and change. The past is of no interest because no one can do anything with it: the present shows more promise; however, the grooves are pretty well established, and the only perspective which promises free expression of manipulative tendencies is the future.

Americans feel under no obligation to conform to the demands of the historical past. They preserve their freedom of action, because they themselves, as the present generation, feel in no way bound to the traditions and bonds passed on from generation to generation. This discontinuity in historical and familial perspective no doubt is in part an expression of the necessary break which occurred when the immigrants left the old country and their past behind. For them, concentration upon the present and the future became a matter of survival.

The expression "Time is money" illustrates the American's attitude toward the present. The present has to be organized, and idleness is not only waste, but harbors the danger of meditation and re-establishment of bonds with the past which may divert energies from the task ahead.

The optimistic perspective towards the future is typically an American outlook on life. The belief in a person's ability to shape his future, and the establishment of conditions which enable people to live in health, have in some way influenced the patient's and the psychiatrist's beliefs in the possibility of therapy. This attitude vividly contrasts with the European tradition, which is characterized by accepting the unalterable facts of a historical past, which in psychiatry was documented by the concern with genetics, constitution, or more recently with existential analysis (173).

GESTALTEN

The term "Gestalt" refers to the views which people take of things and of each other, including the dimensions and organizational details of such perceptions, and the awareness of the contrast between that which is observed and its background. Though "Gestalt" is a concept which denotes the perceptual organization of impressions and the arrangement of information within the observer, its influence upon the shape of man-made object systems and the nature of human relations is far-reaching. If certain features which have been perceived become maximized or minimized because of the spatial arrangement of information, such a distortion in turn is likely to influence subsequent actions. In the study of culture, then, the anthropologist can expect to find the effects of such individual perceptive processes multiplied many hundred times. They are revealed in the material culture as well as in the social relations of a given group of people.

Let us consider first the dimensions of the Gestalten which one encounters in America. One of the features which strike the European is that the people in general are literal-minded, and that the scientists love to measure. In order to measure or to be literal, small pieces of information must be isolated in the perceptual field so that the information becomes ready to be acted upon. It is characteristic of Americans that they tend to isolate rather small Gestalten in their daily work; and bureaucratic practices—that is, emphasis upon administrative details—point towards this end. In contrast to these more concrete considerations, Americans think in terms of large Gestalten when the future is considered. Change and planning always involve larger Gestalten. That which exists is broken down into small pieces, but that which is not yet is envisaged in liberal and oversized dimensions. When an American is frustrated, cornered, or ill at ease, he tends to talk about or be concerned with small details.

Considering next the organization of the Gestalten, be they big or small, we find that the organization of object systems is worked out in great detail and with the same care as the overall picture, if the object is practical and has a functional application. Details of machinery, for example, are worked out to the smallest detail. In contrast, pure ornaments which have only an aesthetic value are disregarded. Likewise quantifiable aspects are worked out much better than qualifiable aspects. The organization of thought as illustrated in philosophy or the organization of feeling as indicated by artistic expression is valued less than the organization of administrative details or of problems of engineering. In science basic problems are neglected in favor of applied fields (35).

The level of complexity varies with the area of endeavor. The European traditionally reproaches the American for his simplicity and his low level of complexity, but it must be borne in mind that in America simplification is carried through until action becomes possible. The Gestalten of American thought are always subordinated to action. In Europe complexity in terms of thought or feeling can exist without ever being subjected to reality testing (109).

The American loves external change and contrasts. Goods are displayed in windows, and contrasting effects are used to catch the eye. Yearly the automotive industry produces new models which by and large show little change in fundamental design except for "face-lifting" around the grill. The variability of things or persons lies in the make-up rather than in the structure of the core. The same contrast which exists in the realm of shape and color is found in temporal matters. Sudden change of occupation, abandonment of a place of residence, speeding up or slowing down in the rate of production, are all events which produce in the human being the effect of contrast. Abrupt transitions and sudden acceleration and deceleration must thus be viewed as a figure-ground contrast along a temporal coordinate.

PROCESSES

"Process" is a term which denotes an observer's comparison of findings over a period of time. The concept of process implies that changes take place along a temporal coordinate and that a scientist who observes and measures certain events is able to relate his findings at various times by a theory of causality or some other theory of relatedness. Therefore, in order to understand change the scientist must be able to fixate his data at any given moment, assuming, of course, that during the period of observation no further change will occur. Such static fixation of data gives information about the structure of events—that is, the arrangement and interconnection of various features— with the help of spatial coordinates and with omission of temporal coordinates. Comparison of such fixations at various intervals thus reintroduces the time coordinate. It must be borne in mind, however, that the human being is at no time able to achieve the same complexity and accuracy in both spatial and temporal analysis. If he emphasizes structure it is at the expense of process, and if he emphasizes process, he will neglect some spatial configurations.

In social relations the scientist cannot make use of any particular instrument which would allow him either to fixate his data or to record changes over a very small or very large time interval, relative to the time scale of the observer. The instruments used are essentially the naked eye and naked ear of the observer; his data are his personal impressions. The scientific universe is therefore limited essentially by the nature of the human recording instrument. Inasmuch as the human organism is a bad timekeeper, it is quite obvious that in the infancy of social sciences the explorer went about to investigate spatial or hierarchical, rather than temporal, connections of events. Only recently have social processes drawn the attention of anthropologists, psychologists, sociologists, and psychiatrists.

The significant difference between the social and the physical sciences is the fact that the physical sciences use recording instruments which fixate the data. Two distinct steps are therefore evident: measurement first, evaluation second. In social science the observation and the evaluation are done in the same step without the aid of instruments. Hence distortions may occur because the social scientist has to act simultaneously as a recording instrument and as an evaluating scientist. Therefore, serving in such a dual capacity, his observation of social processes is necessarily subjectivistic. The human being is able to record changes if they occur within a matter of seconds or weeks. As soon as the time interval becomes too small, as for example a fraction of a second, or too large, for example a decade, the human instrument will not be able to follow the change. Whenever we talk about social process, we must bear these limitations in mind; but knowing these shortcomings, the understanding of social or interpersonal processes may prove helpful not only in psychotherapy but also in planning those conditions which may make for healthier living.

All of us are aware of the existence of social change. However, there exist inherent difficulties in recording and conceptualizing social events. In order to facilitate the understanding of change as it applies to human behavior, the concept of velocity and the concept of rate of change have to be introduced. These terms are borrowed from physics, and the justification for such a procedure may be seen in the fact that the human being walks, talks, and writes at a certain speed. Comparable to physical action, mental actions can be said to possess temporal characteristics. Also one can visualize the speed with which a boy wins a girl, or a speaker convinces his audience, as being a vector quantity in the sphere of interpersonal relations. And last but not least, the speed with which a rumor travels, a panic spreads, and a social reform gets under way, can all be conceived of as velocities of social processes. In Newton's laws of motion, velocity is defined as rate of change of position; it is a vector quantity and therefore has magnitude and direction; the rate of change of these velocities is termed acceleration and deceleration. There seems to be no reason which would stand in the way of applying such highly useful physical concepts to the understanding of intrapersonal and interpersonal phenomena. However, measurement of social processes has to proceed along different lines from those customary in physics.

Applying these notions of process to the understanding of our contemporary scene, we find that Americans, in general, do things fast. Decisions are made with ease, organizations are founded and dissolved without hesitation, and administrative rules and regulations are readily scrapped or amended. Industrial production is fast, and industry is able to change over and retool if different models are needed. While one can say that the velocities of overt behavioral processes in America are probably on the fast side of the scale, the thinking processes show probably a slower rate. It is quite obvious that we get on difficult ground when we talk about the velocity of thinking processes because we are unable to measure thinking directly; inference is all that is possible. However, another observation pertinent to America can be clearly substantiated: the acceleration and deceleration of behavioral processes is considerable. Human relations are quickly initiated and easily dissolved; industrial enterprises mushroom up out of nowhere, and if they do not produce a satisfactory return, are quickly abandoned. Participants at a social gathering will immediately call one another by their first names; in spite of this familiarity, however, they may part a few moments later without saying good-bye. This behavior shows abrupt transition from familiarity to utter detachment, without concern with the transition. To the European the shock experienced by this social abruptness is comparable to that felt when a moving car comes to a sudden emergency stop.

Again, the lack of transition and the abruptness of acceleration and deceleration of social processes are accentuated by the frequent change in social aims. For example, a person is a stranger until he is identified as a prospective buyer, whereupon he is showered with courtesy and friendliness; as soon as the contract is signed, he is immediately relegated again to the status of a complete stranger. Immediate goals are flexibly defined and may be quickly replaced, depending upon the occasion. The foreign observer thus receives a superficial impression of inconsistency and discontinuity; it is his way to express his bewilderment when participating in events, the velocities of which are either faster or slower than the rate to which he is accustomed.

The American tends to quantify. The American scientist is a measurer, and in daily life people tend to list numbers or quote figures in terms of prices or dimensions of things. Quantification is considered the only evidence of truth, and this tendency permeates commerce and public life in general. However, quantification does not extend to the realm of intrapersonal experience. In America the intensity with which emotions are experienced and expressed seems to be at the lower end of the scale, and little attention is paid to feelings and thought. In other words, quantification in America is a process which applies to action rather than to intrapersonal experiences, and if one wishes to include distinctness of goals and direction of efforts as other criteria of quantification, one can state that immediate goals are clearly defined and that immediate action cues, necessary for practical implementation, are explicit and obvious. In contrast, action which is still in the blueprint stage is treated in an indistinct and vague way; Americans rarely commit themselves to any course of future action, inasmuch as such commitment might handicap the flexibility of future adjustment. From the level of national policy—for example, the Monroe Doctrine—to the behavior of the individual, this trend is apparent. Statements referring to future action are often so vague that possible hints are understandable to members of the in-group only.

INTEGRATION

The term "integration" refers to the processes of central codification within an individual organism; it denotes the effort of a person to organize the information derived from apparently heterogeneous experiences. Depending upon the culture, people tend to integrate experiences around either spatial or temporal coordinates; in other words, people will tend to emphasize either structure or process. It is obvious that the manner in which an individual attempts to integrate past experiences will influence future actions. Americans seem to integrate experience around a temporal axis, while some Europeans, in contrast, attempt to integrate around spatial coordinates. The consideration of process in the life of Americans is manifested in the constant awareness of the future, as if the future had already arrived. People plan at the age of twenty for their future retirement, and having this temporal evolution in mind they are deeply concerned with problems of development; children's agencies and bureaus, preventive medicine, the emphasis upon learning all testify to this end. The European, in contrast, is more concerned with purity of style and structure, at any one given moment, than with the nature of change and process. Likewise the European is more interested in being rather universal in his skills; he attempts to coordinate as many features in his life as possible, giving an outward impression of complexity. A European individual with a primarily spatial orientation can consider many factors because he does not assume that change will occur. In contrast, the American's orientation towards process and time limits his attention at any one given moment to fewer factors, and he becomes fascinated by the anticipation of change.

Readiness for change means that the organism must be prepared for action. This we have termed the alarm reaction (148). It is quite obvious that the American population, and patients in particular, exhibit more signs of anxiety than their European contemporaries.

The frequency of manifest signs of anxiety in America is related to the public tolerance of anxiety. This statement appears at first paradoxical. On the one hand, Americans are supposed to strive for complete mastery of their emotions, while on the other hand, we observe that there exists a great tolerance for signs of anxiety in America. The reader need only be reminded that psychiatrists, social workers, and psychologists are constantly talking about anxiety. Movies, television, and advertising are geared to provoke anxiety in the public, and at social gatherings the European is impressed by the display of signs of anxiety. Therefore, we can conclude that the display of signs of anxiety is a feature which is accepted by Americans as long as the display remains implicit and is not verbalized. In America anxiety becomes almost institutionalized. It gives content and substance to the person who has little feeling, and it alerts the individual to forthcoming change. Only the alerted individual can cope quickly and effectively with the changing conditions of his surroundings. Though the European may interpret these features as insecurity, he must be reminded of the fact that such a state of constant alarm is necessary for people who are geared for action, and the reader need only be reminded of the rush and hurry of American life to fully appreciate the meaning of alarm. In Europe, Europeans are much less in a state of alarm because change is not anticipated, though it may occur. The European is much less geared to action; his emphasis is on thoughts and feelings. Since he is capable of an intense inner life, without an externally corresponding stimulation, he does not need to rely as much upon anxiety as a motivating force. Furthermore, since his life is built upon the complexity of thought and feeling, rather than upon the efficiency of action, he also has at his disposal a variety of mental mechanisms which neutralize or hide overt signs of anxiety.

In returning to our previous considerations, it might be said that in a European setting, events are best understood by a structural scheme with spatial coordinates. In America, in contrast, individual and cultural events are better encompassed with the help of a system which is processal in nature with emphasis on temporal coordinates. The American culture is dynamically oriented towards movement and change, while the European culture is essentially static with emphasis on the refinement of the already existing features. Both culture and individuals are geared to these different tasks, and events have to be understood within this general framework.

A PERSPECTIVE OF AMERICAN THERAPY

After this brief theoretical discussion of some general principles which seem to be characteristic of the American scene we shall investigate whether such generalizations are likely to hold true also for the psychiatric scene. To answer this question we once again send our foreign traveler to observe the American psychiatrist in action. Calling on a psychiatrist for the first time, he is struck by the spaciousness, comfort, and luxury of the office suite. Comfortable chair and couch are his equipment, and in addition he may possess an examination room which he uses for neurological examinations. The waiting room is comfortable and cheerful, equipped with a variety of the most recent journals and magazines. Offices are frequently soundproofed, and the luxuriousness of decor reflects upon the status of the physician. Everything is arranged to insure the comfort of both patient and doctor; it is in step with the general treatment of any customer, client, or patient within the American scene.

The American psychiatrist's perspective toward the future is the basis upon which psychotherapy rests. Organization towards the future is the topic to which psychotherapy is dedicated. The concept that "time is money" has made out of therapy an income-producing activity. On the one hand it enables the psychiatrist to make a better living and compels him toward a successful organization of time and practice, while on the other hand the patient treats the money he spends in therapy as an investment which promises returns in the future. We mentioned above the lack of transitions and the suddenness of change in the American pattern of living; we find this same feature in psychotherapy. The patient may terminate therapy with ease, and the psychiatrist may discharge a patient from the carefully guarded hospital environment into the unguarded surroundings of the city without questioning the procedure. Suddenness, abruptness, and unpredictability to the point of shock are accepted as universal features in American life; they profoundly influence psychiatric practices in the United States.

The orientation of the American psychiatrist leans towards large Gestalten as far as temporal matters are concerned, and small Gestalten where structural patterns are involved. The analyst, for example, works out the small Gestalt of a patient's individual perception and memories in great detail even if these are extremely remote from the needs of daily life. But he likewise tends to emphasize interpersonal processes and is far more interested in the manipulation of his patient than his European colleagues. Terms such as "the total personality" or "total adjustment" bear witness of the larger Gestalten considered when processes are the focal point of interest.

If one looks at the topics which are discussed in various forms of therapy, one frequently meets the word "adjustment." One encounters an emphasis upon engineering and applied problems and a neglect of aesthetic and philosophical considerations. The level at which interpretations are given is as simple as possible. The interpretations are geared to practical and workable solutions, i.e., action. In the field of psychiatry, therefore, we find once again the tendency towards simplification and emphasis upon detail because intrapersonal processes are subordinate to subsequent action. The importance of action in American life influences psychiatric thinking, and all psychiatrists are aware of the manipulating tendencies of the patient and of themselves; here affairs have to be handled and managed, while in the European scene stress is placed on experience. The American patient comes in order to get better control of himself and life, while the European, in contrast, will consult a psychiatrist because he feels he does not obtain satisfactory gratification from his present mode of living.

The tendency of the scientist to measure has penetrated psychiatric thinking in America. Attempts to verify therapeutic results by objective criteria at the expense of the subjective feeling of improvement on the part of the patient, which after all is the thing that really matters, may be cited as illustration. Therapy is oriented around process, and a prolonged chipping away at matters of the past, to unearth the detailed structure of the patient's personality, is a feature which is emphasized less and less in American psychotherapy. The quantifiable and processal aspects of social interaction predominate in American psychiatry, a tendency which is reflected in such procedures as the plan for therapy which states predetermined goals and predetermined estimates of time. The original European orientation of therapy toward structure has been gradually changed in America to an orientation toward process. Things have to be done fast in America, and therefore therapy has to be "brief" (3).

Integration of American personalities obviously occurs around a temporal coordinate. It is generally accepted that emotions have a fleeting quality, that personality factors are subject to change; consistency of character is not expected, and display of intense and consistent emotions is avoided. If such a display should occur, its expression is accompanied by guilt. The American cherishes in his personality first and foremost the ability to adapt to changing conditions of life, and consistent and intense emotions would defeat this purpose. Therapy in turn has to serve this purpose; it has become a method to ensure the patient's integration into the American scene. But because of the great speed of things, the essence of therapeutic procedures in America should consist of giving the patients enough time to integrate their experiences. And because of the emphasis on appearance and "wrappings" rather than upon the core of things, the patient needs therapists who emphasize the core. Essentially one may state that therapy has to provide that which the culture does not provide. And in America, with its emphasis upon adjustment, it is experience which the patient needs.

6 · COMMUNICATION AND THE SYSTEM OF CHECKS AND BALANCES: An Anthropological Approach

By Jurgen Ruesch and Gregory Bateson

THE AMERICAN SCENE

EUROPEANS looking at America from across the Atlantic are frequently puzzled and disoriented by American mechanisms of decision. They wonder, for example, whether there is such a thing as an American foreign policy and whether the Secretary of State's word is a binding expression of such policies—if such policy exists. They ask what is the difference between one American political party and another and hope to understand the enigma by equating American parties with the Right and Left of the European political scene. And when, for the moment, they feel satisfied that such an understanding is possible, they are again thrown back into confusion by the blurred quality of American political utterance. From where they sit, it looks as though American officials lacked not only clarity but also forthrightness. During the war, Europeans longed—albeit unrealistically—to hear President Roosevelt speak like Churchill. But had he so spoken, they would have wondered: will his words be later negated by Congress as, historically, happened to Woodrow Wilson?

So much for the distant view. When the European finds himself in America, actually participating in processes of American decision as a member, say, of some committee, he is no less disoriented. It seems to him that no member of a committee quite dares to speak his mind and that the committee as a whole is excessively cautious about any flat statements of its position and policy. And this mysterious caution in the committee room is made still more mysterious by the fact that when Americans are not acting within some organizational framework, they seem to be remarkably—even shockingly—forthright in their utterance. Educated and sensitive Americans in informal conversation will ride roughshod over discriminations of thought to which the European would attach great importance, and yet the same individuals will accurately savor the finest nuances of implicit meaning in an organizational memorandum which has been deliberately written to be as nearly flavorless as possible.

For the sake of vivid presentation, these paradoxes are here described as they appear to the stranger from another culture; but to Americans, of course, these phenomena are not mysterious but either imperceptible or "natural." Sometimes an American may regret the necessity for pulling his punches in political life, sometimes he may be proud of his forthright utterances in an informal context, but in general this contrast is one of which he is rarely aware; and when he notices the discrepancy, it scarcely occurs to him that any alternative might be conceivable. He will see the more uncompromising political pronouncements of a European politician as fanaticism and certainly as politically unwise; while the European's discrimination and sensitivity in the handling of informal relations will appear to an American as a nicety by no means to be admired.

We ask—what are the actual relationships, formal and informal, which are expressed and perpetuated in these characteristics of American communication? Broadly, it seems that the American political scene differs from the European in this respect— that the policies of an American political party are limited from within by the divergent views of its own members, while a European party is controlled by the external existence of opposing parties with contrasting ideologies. A European leader is relatively sure of support from the members who are behind him and relatively sure of uniformity of opinion in the group which he leads. So far as his followers are concerned, he can go to any extreme in the statement of their shared opinions or in actions based upon these opinions. Those who do not agree with him will not be members of his party but will have attached themselves to the party of his opponents. It is the existence of this opposing party which will prevent his party from moving too rapidly in the directions which their ideology would indicate.

In contrast, the American parties are not divided along sharp lines of ideological contrast. They may, and often do, attempt to criticize each other in ideological terms, and on certain issues and at certain times the Republican and Democratic parties may be divided so that it would look as though the ideological issues might be summarized in terms such as "left" and "right." But any such summary would actually do violence to the facts. Within either party ideological contrasts may be observed at least as great as any of the contrasts between them.

The leader of an American party has the problem of maintaining integration in a group characterized by diversity of opinions on matters about which he must make decisions and utter opinions. Whenever he speaks, each utterance is a trial balloon, and he continually watches those behind him to see how far he can go. In conventional psychiatric terms, he is engaged in "reality testing"; in the terminology of the theories which are here proposed, he is asking an implicit question about his own statements referring to a communication about communication: he is asking, "What effect will my utterance have upon relations between my supporters and myself?" He is, also, *ipso facto*, making implicit metacommunicative statements about his own position and stock of information: "I lack certain information about my relationship with my followers"; "I feel a need for this information"; "I am deferring to the (to me unknown) opinion of my followers"; and so on.

So much for the description of the phenomena. It is now our task to express these observations in a more systematized manner, and we do so by introducing the concept of the system of internal checks and balances and the system of external oppositional control. The European viewpoint would be appropriately represented by the system of external control, while the American approach is better exemplified in the system of internal checks. Let us now consider the nature of these concepts.

THE SYSTEM OF INTERNAL CHECKS AND BALANCES

Let us consider an American political party or the American form of government, including legislative, executive, and judicial branches, or a welfare organization, or an American university. All of these organizations have features in common which can be conceptualized in a description not intended to fit any specific case but only to illustrate the principles involved:

The organization is run by a team, the official representative of which may be called the executive. The latter usually has a staff of administrative assistants who keep in touch with all the other members and departments of the organization. The actions of the executive are checked by the other members of the team, composed of committee members and technical advisers. The executive, the committee members, and the technical advisers divide their duties as follows: the technical advisers are the ones who are most consciously aware of the state of affairs; they are responsible for the collection and interpretation of data relevant to the activities of the organization; they are the scientists, technicians, researchers, and theorists of the organization. The committee members, on the other hand, are the representatives of pressure groups. They represent the constituent groups and hence have the function of checking and counterchecking the whole system; by and large they lack technical knowledge, but possess the "common horse sense" of politicians. The executive, in turn, is the one who keeps the committees in balance and who represents the whole group in relations with the outside world. It is his job to be aware of the tensions within the organization, and he must try to remedy disturbances which might break up the coalition. In most American organizations, if large enough, it is customary to have also a sample of the outside world represented within the organization. This representation is found in the board of supervisors or board of trustees, who represent the citizenship or membership at large. They act as a check upon the pressure groups as represented by the committee members and personified in the executive. If all groups interact appropriately, the success of the organization is assured. If interaction is unsuccessful, a new coalition must be formed until the organization becomes balanced once again.

The reader will recognize that the functioning of the system of checks is based upon the interrelation of smaller units which, through mutual cooperation, form a larger unit. Each entity acts as a speed-up or brake mechanism for the whole system, thus regulating the rate or direction of change of the over-all system. The system of checks is based upon self-regulation, and it can function relatively independently of other systems because of its circular characteristics. The major system as such is not solidly knit and represents really an envelope for the various sub-systems. Leadership in such an organization is not concentrated in a single man with absolute executive power; usually there is a group or committee composed of a number of equals, which as an aggregate has more power than the single person at the head of the organization who personifies the system. Public opinion attributes power to him, while in reality such a man depends upon the power given to him by various groups. The men with the real power may be found in the persons of committee members or in technical advisers; or perhaps they may not even be officially connected with the organization. If any of these people become too powerful, the extreme sanction for too great an assumption of power by one single man consists of expulsion from the pressure group and hence exclusion from any actual or prospective gains. The expelled individual will need a long time to rebuild the power he has lost, and the punishment received can be viewed as a reprimand for non-conformance with the rules of the game.

The problems of administration are continually posed and resolved in terms of competitive strivings for expansion and power by various groups, but none will subscribe to an agreement which would allow any one group to be in power without limitations in terms of time, rights, and privileges. In the struggle for power, persons with social or personal goals form a pressure group and try to obtain power not in ideological but in practical terms, and any one group may enlist the help of other groups of different ideologies in order to obtain power. It is characteristic of systems of this sort that at all levels, both groups and subgroups lack uniformity of opinion. Rather, each group represents a spectrum or diversity of opinion, and the integrating factors are not ideological or even matters of broad policy; instead the group is integrated around the overlapping of purposes. In such a system, the structure of the parts is a repetition of the structure of the whole. The nation, the political party, and the pressure groups within the party are alike in that each of these entities is characterized by a diversity of opinion; and this feature obtains in the structure of the American family and in the personality of the American individual.

To summarize the characteristics of the system of internal checks and balances one can state that:

(a) It is composed of heterogeneous elements which are allowed to maintain their heterogeneity.

(b) It has a circular character in which change, correction, and self-regulation are implied.

(c) It attempts to exist in relative isolation from other systems.

(d) Its integration occurs in terms of shared purposes rather than broad opinions or ideologies.

THE SYSTEM OF EXTERNAL OPPOSITIONAL CONTROLS

The system of internal checks will stand out clearly when compared with the system of oppositional control. The latter is more characteristic of European cultures, and perhaps of those special areas of America where English, French, and Spanish modes of organization have persisted. Indeed, in some instances it is to be expected that the two types of systems will coexist.

In the system of oppositional control a number of entities of about equal force maintain their separateness and curb each other. The regulation of the dynamics of the over-all system and of its rates and direction of change is determined by the entities which oppose each other. In such systems, leadership and administration are handled quite differently from the ways in which an American organization is managed. The European leader can rely upon the homogeneity of the group behind him, and he can be sure that those who disagree with the ideology of the party will be members of opposing parties—not unwilling followers whom he must placate within his own organization. Similarly, the allegiance of the members will be differently based. In nineteenth-century England, Gilbert and Sullivan's *Iolanthe* caricatured this situation:

> That every boy and every gal
> That's born into the world alive
> Is either a little Liberal
> Or else a little Conservative.

As Gilbert saw it, political action was determined by allegiance and status, and the political differences between individuals were an expression of deep-seated trends of the personality. He could hardly have made such a remark about Republicans and Democrats in America, where political action is governed by sharing of goals and opportunity rather than by ideology and personality structure.

Within the system of oppositional control homogeneity and allegiance would lead to a fast-moving, almost revolutionary organization, unless checked by other organizations, similarly constructed but with different and conflicting ideologies. Moreover, the fact that the leader can rely upon the homogeneity of the members is much more likely to lead to the formation of a single authoritarian hierarchy within the party. Inasmuch as the members are self-committed to allegiance, they cease to function as corrective forces. The leader need not placate his supporters, and therefore he himself is ex officio the authority. In the words of Louis XIV, *"L'état, c'est moi."* Historically speaking, the French Revolution was a significant break in the system of oppositional control, and indeed France after much experimentation has never achieved any stable solution to the problem of integrating oppositional forces.

This problem can perhaps only be solved if two seemingly

conflicting conditions are met: (a) a balance of power must exist in the population; and (b) a sufficient majority must be maintained in the seat of governmental power so that decision is not hampered by discord. But these conditions are—especially today—difficult to meet, and there is always some danger that action may be paralyzed by balanced discord in the seat of government. This paralysis occurs from time to time in the parliaments of western Europe (Weimar Republic, England, France) and may lead to popular discontent and frustration. In the extreme case, an avalanche of popular sentiment may result in irreversible change, placing a single individual or party in absolute power. In some European countries the function of validating the power of the party which for the moment has a majority in parliament is assigned to a non-partisan referee such as the King of England or the President of the French Republic.

There are, in fact, three types of leaders in a system of oppositional controls: (a) the non-partisan authority, the king or monarch, whose function is described above; (b) the leader of a homogeneous group or party whose authority within the party is rarely challenged; and (c) the dictator who may arise in such a system by riding a single party into absolute power. In this case, the former leader of a subgroup comes to occupy the position of monarch without giving up his partisan allegiance. The sanctions for nonconformists in this system are rather definite and explicit; in case of a violation of rules, in-group status is lost and the nonconforming person is removed from office, and usually becomes isolated.

These homogeneous, tightly knit authoritarian groups compete with each other, be it in the form of business, politics, or sports. Whenever one such system is removed, the equilibrium of power is disturbed. This fact is exemplified in the political role of Germany in central and western Europe. All nations feared and fought Germany, but apparently Europe does not function properly without it, and now as in 1918 a strengthening of Germany is advocated by its former enemies.

If we now summarize the characteristics of the system of external oppositional controls, we arrive at the following conclusions:

(a) The system consists of homogeneous elements. All deviant elements are eliminated and have to form new groups.

(b) The system has a hierarchical structure; change and correction occur only under external pressure or internal disruption.

(c) The system cannot exist in isolation, but instead is dependent for control of its homogeneity upon the existence of other systems which are different, but which are themselves homogeneous. This external pressure supplies the necessary motivation for self-control, results in differentiation within the assigned limits, and justifies concentration of power at the head of the unit.

COMMUNICATION IN THE SYSTEM OF CHECKS

The description of the systems of internal checks and external controls can be viewed as a statement of a culture scout, who wishes to arrange certain information he has gathered about people in a comprehensive and orderly manner. The scientific interpretation of the word "system," bearing essentially upon events located inside the observer, has to be complemented by another meaning of the word "system" which refers to information inherent in the population studied. "System" as used in this latter sense bears upon the mode of adaptation and communication of the people and constitutes, so to speak, a code with which a participant is enabled to communicate. Such a code includes not only the symbolic systems of a given culture but contains communications about communication. In each culture the participants communicate not only content, but also instructions on how to interpret a given message. Such communications about communication can be described scientifically by neutral observers in terms of systems; the citizens of the communities involved, however, apply this knowledge in daily communication without being aware of its existence. The double meaning of the concept of system, first as explicit knowledge for the observer, next as implicit cue for the participant, can be illustrated with the topic of authority.

THE INTERPRETATION OF GOVERNMENTAL AUTHORITY IN THE SYSTEM OF CHECKS

Let us consider for a moment American conditions of about one or two hundred years ago. A wide open continent, unlimited resources in terms of land and raw materials on the one hand, and untamed nature and hostile Indians on the other hand, necessitated an inclusive cooperative attitude of its settlers, who in frontier situations had known each other for a brief period only. To get the most out of a group of people who need each other and who want to cooperate but who do not trust each other can be conceived as the basic need which underlies the system of checks; this idea is implicitly held by every American. Under the conditions prevalent some hundred years ago traditional positions of authority were unsuitable, while at the same time concentration of power into one hand became an absolute necessity, always with the understanding that at any moment such delegated executive power could be withdrawn and given to somebody else. The need for flexibility to meet unforeseen emergencies and the relatively fast pace of events which to the naïve observer may have appeared as discontinuity, favored the establishment of social equality and the maintenance of diversified ways to acquire power.

Flexibility and change are essentially related to metropolitan industrial as well as to nomadic life, resulting in delegated, functional authority. In contrast, authority as a personality feature develops where there is a preponderance of agriculture, and where people settle in small villages. Here we find the typical hierarchical and patriarchal structure in which the division of labor, distribution of power, and assignment of authority can remain the same throughout a lifetime. Though superficially the same, the head man of an American organization is not to be confused with a European patriarch. The American executive personifies an organization and its multiple and conflicting interests, but he really has not an authoritarian role. The position of American president is somehow typical; while on the one hand he possesses more power than any kind of dictator, he is, on the other hand, checked constantly by Cabinet members, Congress, courts, and public opinion; his tenure in office is limited. In America the President expresses in some way the opinion of the Cabinet and other advisers who represent the various factions of the party in power. It is well to remember that each of the two major American political parties is made up of individuals ranging from extreme conservatives to extreme liberals. These heterogeneous elements act as brakes and accelerators within each of the two parties. The foreigner frequently misunderstands that the opposition between the Democratic and Republican parties is essentially a non-ideological competition for power. The ideological platforms are selected prior to the time of election and are purely instrumental in character. In contrast, in the system of controls conservatives would be found in one and liberals in another party. The cabinet would express the opinion of the prime minister, and the ideologies of the government would express the consistent and inflexible opinion of its leaders.

THE SHAPING OF PERSONALITIES IN THE SYSTEM OF CHECKS

Premises pertaining to the superpersonal system of internal checks are present in every American, and therefore these premises are an integral part of his personality. Each individual's knowledge about the "American way of life" contains the cues with which a message can be interpreted. For example, the American personality will be inclined to tolerate heterogeneous elements in its own behavior; it allows itself to change opinions, occupations, wives or husbands, places of residence, and the like, always aware of the fact that such actions are permissible if they improve the well-being within the socially approved limits. Such adaptive actions can be summarized under the heading of independence, self-sufficiency, moderation, collaborative cooperation with others, and readiness for change. An individual who acts according to the prevailing system will interpret incoming and send outgoing messages with these directives unconsciously in mind. Then he is "well adjusted."

Conflict, be it intrapersonal, interpersonal, or with the environment, must be handled. The American believes in solutions and alternatives, compromise and change. Action and implementation are highly valued, and that part of the personality which Freud referred to as ego becomes the center of all psychological concerns. In contrast, the European with his more fatalistic outlook believes much less in action, prefers to accept the unavoidable, and therefore is more concerned with personality aspects such as the "id" or the "superego." The European makes an attempt at integrating and synthesizing heterogeneous elements within his personality structure; differences are accepted as existing between people, but not in one person; differentiation and complexity developed in one area of the personality are carried over to the other areas, at the expense of readiness for change. Such striving for wholeness and universality is exemplified in the ideal of humanistic education. Unification, however, seems not to be possible without some coercion. Control has to be exerted in terms of a variety of mechanisms which are intended to keep the inhibited drives under control. Likewise the European is not allowed to change opinions, occupations, or places of residence. Instead, the individual has to move along certain grooves determined by class, caste, and occupation, from which there is no escape. Stepping over these boundaries entails fighting all those whose territory has been trespassed upon, and in absence of any readiness for compromise, the conflict, intrapersonal as well as interpersonal, usually becomes rather severe.

Let us now compare these large-scale events with happenings on an individual level. When we consider events happening in America on a group or cultural level, we talk about a political system of internal checks and balances; when we consider events on an individual level, we speak of action and ego psychology. "Superego" and "id" are treated in the individual system as if they were pressure groups which had to be appeased by the executive, the "ego." The latter is perceived as the real self. In contrast, the system of external oppositional control is reflected on an intrapersonal level in "id" and "superego" psychology. Within such a system the individual experiences the "superego" as an element which controls the "id." The real self is identified primarily with the "id" and to a lesser degree with the "superego." Clashes between "superego" and "id" are accepted and valued as the essence of the self. And while awareness and enjoyment of conflict characterizes the European personality, compromise and smoothness are valued by the American personality.

FAMILY STRUCTURE IN THE SYSTEM OF CHECKS

The system of checks and balances which seems characteristic for American political organizations has its counterpart in the styling of interpersonal relations within the family circle. The American family is a unit with imperfectly defined leadership and a spectrum of opinions. Neither parent is in a position of recognized final authority. It often happens that one parent is more active in making decisions than the other; or one parent may be more important than the other as the link between the family and the rest of the community. But a parent who takes over such special functions is still not a final authority or spearhead for the family unit. He or she is not in a position to make decisions and be sure that the other members will accept and support the decision. Rather, the outstanding parent must overtly act as though he or she were orchestrating a diversity of opinions—and must perform this function not with a silent baton, but playing actually in the orchestra, exerting an integrating influence only by his or her contribution to the total sequence of sound. It follows that the would-be leader's contribution, to be effective, must have many elements in common with the sounds and themes produced by the other players. If one parent is acting as leader, he or she can only influence the others if they in turn are able to hear a proportion of their own sentiment echoed in the leader's voice; while reciprocally for the leader, the sentiments and views of the followers are in some sort his sounding board determining the direction which he can take and limiting how far he can go.

Americans accept hokum on the part of their leaders with great tolerance. It is as if the avoidance of confrontation led to a new form of shrewdness and a new form of sincerity. To European eyes the dispenser of hokum is simply a charlatan and an object for contempt; in American eyes, his dishonesty is negated by the fact that everybody knows that the vocal leader must dilute what he wants to say with a vast mass of what he thinks people want to hear. He must give his audience what they want. Nobody more than half believes him, and he can therefore remain a beloved figure whose deceit is felt to be vaguely benevolent—even therapeutic. The psychological status of these figures is vividly documented in the enormously popular children's stories of the "Wizard of Oz." This glorified huckster, even after his deceits have been exposed, gives a heart to the Tin Woodsman, a brain to the Scarecrow, and courage to the Cowardly Lion. To Dorothy, the heroine, he gives the faith which will enable her to return to Kansas.

In the continuous process, where all contribute to the integration of the group, any flat statement of disagreement is dangerous, but Americans can "agree to disagree." This phrase usually denotes more than it says. Literally it would imply that each of the two persons agrees to the fact that the other has a different opinion from himself, but in addition when they agree to disagree they acknowledge that in spite of the differences of opinion they have a common goal. At a minimum, they have a common goal in avoiding continued argument and strife, but usually they are thinking of still more positive goals, and it is the explicit or implicit appeal to these goals which is the cement whereby diverse opinions are united into a system of checks. Americans avoid confrontation and statement of position and the stressing of difference which would occur in many European cultures. Avoidance of confrontation is associated with purposiveness and orientation toward the future, while compromise and readiness to get together with the aim of a shared purpose break any possible deadlock and bridge differences of opinion.

Everybody in the family group acts as a check upon the other members. Roles are constantly changing, and therefore the American child faces certain difficulties related to the delineation of his identity. For example, in the father's voice there are overtones of the mother's sentiments; and in the mother's voice when she addresses the child there are overtones of agreement with the child. And yet, in terms of human reality, transcending all such cultural peculiarities, a child is a separate entity living in his own private world with his own system of goals and aspirations. If he lives in an American family he will, whenever his parents speak, hear his own aspirations woven into a system which is not his. His opportunities for discovering the facts of human individuality are thus blurred whenever one parent echoes the sentiments of the other. Self-identification develops through the observation that the self is different from other people and that people are different from each other. But the American child has a more complicated path to compass. On the one hand he must discover that he is himself different; and on the other hand, he must learn a way of life in which he has to obliterate his own individuality. If he does not learn this he will be continually frustrated in a world which operates under the premise of presumed resemblances.

Through his family experiences, the American child is adequately, even excessively, prepared for membership in a group. He has assimilated the premise that the group exercises moral censorship. The transition from personalized parental authority to subservience to group authority occurs a long time before physical separation from the parents takes place. Assumption of self-censorship in the American personality—or, to use a Freudian term, the development of the "superego"—is therefore the result of an integrated group experience rather than being based upon a direct identification with, for example, the father. In contrast, the English child is more prepared to accept the leader of a group as a parental substitute or, if he finds himself in the position of leader with a role that focuses the eyes of a group upon him, he will adopt a parental attitude toward the group.

In a vast majority of cases, the American child passes through a phase of gang membership—i.e., a period in which he is a participating member of a group of age mates existing outside the home. American parents are often keenly conscious of this group as a character-forming influence, alien to their own generation and often alien to their own cultural background. They are probably in error in this evaluation: what really happens is that the child brings to his group membership that precise deference to the idea of the group which was implanted in him by the family constellation. Of relevance at this point is the management of exhibitionism and spectatorship (17). The American parent tends to use his spectatorship to encourage the child toward achievements and self-sufficiency; while the English parent uses exhibitionism—acting as a model and inviting the child's spectatorship—so that the child may learn how to act. It thus happens that in America, exhibitionism is linked with childish themes of dependence and submission; while in England exhibitionism is linked with parental themes of dominance and nurture. It was stated above that the would-be leader in America must overtly show that he is exerting his leadership through his contribution as a participant, so that the group can exert a certain amount of control. In so doing the leader is necessarily in some degree exhibitionistic, and by that token he is in a sense dependent upon the group's approval and submissive to their limiting control.

PSYCHIATRY IN A WORLD OF CHECKS AND BALANCES

Organized psychiatry follows the pattern of the system of checks and balances prevalent in American life. The professional organizations of psychiatrists such as the American Psychiatric Association, the American Psychosomatic Society, and the American Orthopsychiatric Association are organized according to a system of checks in which the internal heterogeneity provides the necessary brakes and corrective mechanisms for the organization. The leadership and members of the policy-making committees represent the various pressure groups. In spite of the differences in focus of professional interests in the various organizations, there is a large proportion of overlapping membership, and the associations do not compete with each other as would be the case if the system followed the pattern of oppositional control. Where the psychiatric schools and orthodoxies are in conflict, as for example in the case of the Freudian and Neo-Freudian schools, the habit of organized dissension was introduced from Europe by Europeans, who were used to the system of oppositional control. Indeed, the gradual influence of America can already be seen in the fact that the various schools are losing their distinctness and becoming more inclusive as the years go by. In other words, even the various psychiatric schools adjust to the prevailing

American system and switch from the organizational characteristics of the system of control to a pattern more in line with the system of checks.

The system of checks and balances can also be found operating in single psychiatric units. In university teaching centers, for example, we find representatives of various schools of therapy; there are the organicists, the mentalists, the social workers, the psychologists, and the occupational therapists working together as teams. The staff and the views of the staff are certainly heterogeneous, and it is the task of the head of the department to maintain heterogeneity as well as a well-functioning unit.

The treatment of authority in such teaching units is remarkable. There is no personal authority, but only functional authority. According to the case, the teacher possesses authority based upon his superior knowledge and skills; but this in turn can be questioned by the pupils and objective evidence demanded. In contrast, the European teacher is usually an exhibitionist, as all European leaders are; he is beyond and safe from all questioning. The American teacher fits into the role of the parent as he is checked by the pupil and watches the first steps taken by the pupil. It is remarkable to see with what security and exhibitionism the American pupil undertakes those first steps in practicing a newly acquired skill. The hesitation with which their European counterparts would proceed to do so is obviously related to the fact that exhibitionism is reserved only for the leaders.

The great American ideal of teamwork dominates academic life and hospital practices. No one remains unchallenged, everyone is corrected and criticized by colleagues, superiors, and inferiors, and little resentment is felt. The dynamic family unit with alternating roles and specialized duties, varying with the circumstances, all sharing a common goal, prepares the professional man for his career.

The system of checks also penetrates therapeutic teamwork. The therapist is definitely an American authority; functional and changeable, the therapist learns as much from his patients as the patients from the therapist. This process of mutual correction is probably the most effective therapeutic agent. The doctor is not only the understanding parent who watches the steps of the child, but he also reminds the patient of the demands of society. In that sense the American therapist helps the patient to fit into the American scene; he acts very much like the board of trustees in a large organization. While the European therapist's goal is to increase the patient's gratification and encourage his narcissistic tendencies, the American therapist's aim is to socialize the patient. This is done by making the patient accept the fact that the group acts as a censor of his actions. Socialization and adjustment are the key words of American therapy. Differences which exist between the patient and his contemporaries are reduced through efforts of therapy; paradoxically this is achieved by making the patient accept the fact that he is different from others; after his acceptance of this difference he no longer feels threatened, and gradually learns to accept the fact that he is like other people. In Europe the converse is true; there the patient is afraid that he is not unique, that he is uncreative, and that he is too much like others. In therapy he learns to accept his similarities with others, and such acceptance then provides the motive for working out his own unique features.

It seems fair to say that the system of checks dominates the American life on a political, group, and individual level. Knowledge of the system of checks provides the individual with the necessary cues to initiate appropriate action and to understand the actions of others. In that sense, awareness of the system of checks constitutes information pertaining to communication about communication—a field which is one of the primary concerns of the psychiatrist.

7 · INFORMATION AND CODIFICATION: A Philosophical Approach

By Gregory Bateson

UP TO this point, this book has been about human beings—specifically, about Americans and about psychiatrists. It has been shown that two types of organized information must be added to psychiatric theory in order to understand the theories and operations of psychiatrists—namely, an understanding of the cultural matrix within which the psychiatrist operates and an understanding of the nature of interaction between persons.

The present chapter and that which follows will attempt to unite these two sorts of additional understanding into a single science so that the phenomena of human culture and personal interaction will take their places in a wider and more abstract theory of communication.[1]

To do this it will be necessary to go back to first principles and to discuss the phenomena of communication as these occur at very low levels of organization, among animals and in the functioning of machines. From this low level, we shall work upward by adding extra degrees of complexity until we again come to speak of entities at a human and cultural level. The total theory

[1] In regard to the cybernetic ideas which are here put forward, I wish to express my indebtedness to the Josiah Macy, Jr., Foundation, which has sponsored a series of conferences on this subject, in all of which I have participated. I also wish to express my special indebtedness to Drs. McCulloch, Wiener, Pitts, Hutchinson, and other members of these conferences whose thinking has deeply influenced my own.

will then be applied in Chapter 10 to a re-examination of some of the theories and statements of American psychiatrists.

THE NATURE OF CODIFICATION

It is necessary first to point out certain general notions about the nature of intrapersonal and neurophysiological processes— notions so general as to be independent of the types of theory which the reader may prefer. The notion of *codification* is, we think, of such a general nature as to be common to all psychological theories, though not always explicit. Whether we favor organicist or mentalist concepts, it is clear that the intrapersonal processes are distinctly different from the events in the external world, and the concept of codification refers to this difference. Using an organicist phrasing, one might say that impulses and showers of impulses traveling in the neural network are the internal reflection or picture of the external events about which the organism is receiving information through his sense organs. Or following mentalist theories, one may say that ideas and propositions (whether verbal or nonverbal) are the translation or reflection of external events. In either theory—organicist or mentalist—internal events are different from external and are reflections or translations of events in the external world. The term used by communications engineers for the substitution of one type of event for another, such that the event substituted shall in some sense stand for the other, is *codification*.

The basic principles upon which information is codified in the brain or mind of human beings are still unknown, but from the external characteristics of human beings and from what communications engineers can tell us, certain generalities are clear.

First, codification must, in the nature of the case, be systematic. Whatever objects or events or ideas internal to the individual represent certain external objects or events, there must be a systematic relationship between the internal and the external, otherwise the information would not be useful. The engineer's term for nonsystematic elements in codification is "noise"; in the presence of too many such random elements there would be no possibility of "decodification"—that is, no possibility of steering the individual's actions in regard to external events. (Strictly there is, of course, no "decodification." Information codified in the form of, for example, neural impulses may guide the organism in its verbal utterances or in action. But these types of output are again codifications or transformations of the neural showers. The information is never translated back into the actual objects to which it refers.)

Second, it is evident that the codification must be such that relationships are preserved. While it is impossible for a man to have inside himself a tree corresponding to the external tree that he perceives, it is possible to have internal objects or events so related to each other that their relations reflect relationships between parts of the external tree. Obviously very profound transformations occur in any codification—and indeed, codification is transformation in the mathematical sense of the word. We may expect, for example, to find in some cases that spatial relations in the external world will be represented by temporal relations in the processes of mind: when the eye scans an object, the shape of the object is certainly transformed into a temporal sequence of impulses in the optic nerve. And in other cases, temporal sequences will be represented as spatial relations in the brain: a memory of past sequences must surely be so codified. But whatever the transformations of codification, information is merely lost unless relations among external events are systematically translated into other relations among the events and processes of the mind (45), (182).

Further, engineers (27) are able to describe several known possible varieties of codification, with which we can compare and contrast what seems to happen in human beings. Broadly there are three important kinds, all of which possibly occur in human mental processes. All three types of codification are also exemplified by various sorts of electronic machinery, and the mechanical examples will be cited to give a more vivid idea of what is meant by codification.

First, there is what the engineers call "digital" codification. This is the method used in the ordinary desk calculating machine, which is made up of interlocking cogs and is essentially a counting mechanism which counts the teeth of the cogs and how many times they rotate in complex interaction. In this type of codification the input already differs very profoundly from the external events about which the machine is "thinking." In fact, for such machines it is necessary to have a human being who will codify the external events in terms of their arithmetical *relations* and feed this codification into the machine in an appropriate manner which defines what problem the machine is to solve.

Second, there is the type of calculating machine which the engineers call "analogic." In these machines the external events about which the machine is to think are represented in the machine by a recognizable model. For example, a wind tunnel is a thinking machine of this kind. In such machines changes in the external system can be represented by corresponding changes in the internal model, and the results of such changes can then be observed. Whether any analogic mechanisms exist in the human central nervous system is exceedingly doubtful, but subjectively we think that we form images of the external world, and these images seem to aid us in our thinking. The nature of these conscious images is, however, obscure, and in any case it is difficult to imagine the operation of any true analogic model in a system such as the central nervous system, which has no moving parts. Apart from the central nervous system, however, there is a possibility that the whole moving body may be used as an analogic component. It is probable, for example, that some people empathize the emotions of others by kinesthetic imitation. In this type of thinking, the body would be an experimental analogue, a model, which copies changes in the other person, and the conclusions from such experimental copying would be derived by the more digital central nervous system which receives proprioceptive cues. It is also certain that human beings often use parts of the external world as analogic models to aid them in solving their own internal problems. Indeed, many patients use the psychotherapist in this way.

Third, there are a few machines which are capable of codifying information in units comparable to what the psychologists call Gestalten (108). An example of such a machine is the recently invented device which reads aloud from printed matter. The machine recognizes the twenty-six letters and makes a different sound for each letter. Further, it recognizes these letters in spite of minor differences between different sorts and sizes of type font, and it also recognizes the same letter regardless of where its image falls upon the screen. In sum, the machine must allow for lateral or vertical displacement on a "retina" and for slight rotational displacement. In achieving this recognition, the machine is doing something very closely comparable to that recognition of Gestalten whereby a human being knows that a square is a square even though it may be of almost any size and presented at any angle. The essential characteristic of such machines is that they can identify formal relations between objects or events in the external world and classify groups of such events according to certain formal categories. A message denoting the presence or absence of an event which fits a certain formal category is then transmitted, possibly by a single signal within the machine. This last possibility of summarizing a complex message in a single "pip" is the advantage which Gestalt codification provides. An enormous economy of communication within the machine can thus be achieved.

A fundamental difference between codification by Gestalten and enumerative digital codification can be illustrated by contrasting codification which occurs in the type of machine which will transmit a half-tone block picture over wire with the type of codification in the process which we call vision. The machine transmits billions of messages. Each message is the presence or absence of a "pip," such presence or absence denoting the presence or absence of a dot in the original half-tone block. The machine is in no way concerned with what the picture represents. On the other hand, a human being looking at such a picture sees it as representing a man, a tree, or what not. The shower of impulses originating in the retina and traveling in the optic nerve is in some ways not unlike the shower of pips transmitted by the machine, but in the brain this neural shower impinges upon a network which has the characteristic of being able to discriminate formal relations within the shower—these formal relations being, in fact, related to those which exist in the original picture. The human being is thus able to categorize large areas of the picture in terms of Gestalten.

The existence of Gestalt processes in human thinking seems to be the circumstance which makes us believe that we are able to think about concrete objects, not merely about relationships. And this belief is further fortified by our use of language, in which substantives and verbs always stand for externally perceived Gestalten. When, however, it is realized that the recognition of Gestalten depends upon the formal relations among external events, then it is evident that thinking in terms of "things" is secondary—an epiphenomenon which conceals the deeper truth that we still think only in terms of relationships. We may summarize the external relationships by constructing Gestalten in our minds, but still it is the relationships in the afferent neural showers which provide the basis for our Gestalten.

The same general truth—that all knowledge of external events is derived from the relationships between them—is recognizable in the fact that to achieve more accurate perception, a human being will always resort to change in the relationship between himself and the external object. If he is inspecting a rough spot on some surface by means of touch, he moves his finger over the spot, thus creating a shower of neural impulses with definite sequential structure, from which he can derive the static shape and other characteristics of the thing investigated. To judge the weight of an object we heft it in the hand, and to inspect a seen object with care we move our eyes in such a way that the image of the object moves across the fovea. In this sense, our initial sensory data are always "first derivatives," statements about *differences* which exist among external objects or statements about *changes* which occur either in them or in our relationship to them. Objects and circumstances which remain absolutely constant relative to the observer, unchanged either by his own movement or by external events, are in general difficult and perhaps always impossible to perceive. What we perceive easily is difference and change—and difference is a relationship.

The Gestalt psychologists have stressed the relations between "figure" and "ground," and while we are not concerned here with the detailed elaboration of Gestalt theory, it is necessary to stress one broad characteristic of the figure-ground phenomenon which must be allowed for in any attempts we may make to understand the codification which occurs in human mental processes. In all figure-ground phenomena, it seems that the perceiver uses the fact that certain end organs are *not* stimulated as a datum for achieving a fuller understanding of those impulses which come from end organs which are stimulated. A human subject, if he places his hand in a closed illuminated box, can tell from neural impulses of warmth or pain originating in his hand that there is illumination, but he cannot decide whether the light comes from a small bright source, or is a general illumination of the box. With his retina, on the other hand, he can immediately tell the difference between general illumination and a small source of light. He does this by combining in the brain the information that certain end organs have been stimulated with the information that certain others were *not*, or were less stimulated. Similarly, as was noted above, in the transmission of a half-tone block the *absence* of pips on wire at a specific moment can be a signal denoting the absence of a dot on the picture. (The mechanical system could as easily have been set up so that the absence of a pip in the wire would denote the presence of a dot in the picture, etc.) This ability of the human brain to use the *absence* of certain afferent impulses in the interpretation of those impulses which do arrive, seems to be a primary condition of the figure-ground phenomenon. We may see the ability to distinguish between general illumination and a small source of light as an elementary form of Gestalt perception.

Further, it would seem that in creating Gestalten the perceiver rules out as irrelevant "ground" a great many impulses which actually impinge upon end organs. The construction of Gestalten would seem to depend upon something like inhibition—a partial negation of certain impulses—which permits the perceiver to attend to those matters which he perceives as "figures."

One of the characteristics of codified information follows from what has been said above, especially from the discussion of the figure-ground hypothesis. This is the fact that information is always *multiplicative*. Every piece of information has the characteristic that it makes a positive assertion and at the same time makes a denial of the opposite of that assertion. The very simplest perception that we can imagine, upon which, for example, the tropisms of protozoa are presumably based, must still tell the organism that there is light in that direction and not light in that other direction. Many pieces of information may be more complex than this, but always the elementary unit of information must contain at least this double aspect of asserting one truth and denying some often undefined opposite. From this it follows that when we have two such "bits" (155) of information the gamut of possible external events to which the information may refer is reduced not to a half, but to a quarter, of the original range; similarly three "bits" of information will restrict the possible gamut of external events to an eighth.

The multiplicative nature of information is illustrated by the game of Twenty Questions. The questioner in this game must, in twenty questions, identify what object the respondent has in mind. The respondent can only answer the questions with "yes" or "no." Every question answered segments the possible range of objects which the respondent might have in mind, and if the questioner plans his questions correctly, in twenty questions he can determine among something over a million objects which one it is that the respondent has in mind ($2^{20} = 1,048,576$). The questioner structures the possible universe of objects with a ramifying system of questions which is what we would call a "codification system," and a very brief trial of the game will give the reader an idea of the difficulties which occur in communication when the two persons do not have precisely similar codification systems—i.e., when the respondent misunderstands the questions. If the game is played strictly according to the rules, there is almost no way of correcting such misunderstandings: the questioner can hardly detect what has happened.

CODIFICATION AND VALUE

Briefly, what we here attempt to argue is that the system of codification and the system of values are aspects of the same central phenomena. The precise relation between the notions of value and information has exercised Occidental philosophers for two thousand years, and a final formulation is not to be expected in this book. It is necessary, however, to strive to make our position clear if we are to study the clash and transmission of values.

We examine first some of the resemblances which seem to link value with codification:

1. The value system and the codification system are alike in that each is a system ramifying through the total world of the individual. The value system, as organized in terms of preference, constitutes a network in which certain items are selected and others passed over or rejected, and this network embraces everything in life. Similarly, it was pointed out in regard to the codification system that all events and objects which present themselves are in some degree classified into the complex system of Gestalten which is the human codification system.

2. A further resemblance springs from the fact that both in the case of codification and in the case of value, the negated class is usually undefined. In the case of preference, a man will say that he likes this or that but will often omit to define the alternatives to which this or that is preferred. Alternatively he may say that he dislikes such and such and will omit to state what he would like better. Similarly in the codification of information human beings discard the ground and observe the figure. People will say that the figure has "meaning" for them; and that that which is preferred or that which is disliked has value as against an undefined background of alternatives.

3. It is well known that the network of value partially determines the network of perception. This is best illustrated by the experiments of Adalbert Ames, Jr., in which a person is made to act in a situation in which he is subject to an optical illusion—i.e., perceives a false Gestalt. Even though he is aware of the illusion, it is almost impossible for him to correct his action

except by many repeated trials. Gradually he learns to correct for the shape which he knows to be real, even though, at first, he cannot see that the objects have this shape. As he achieves correction, his image of the objects changes and he begins to see them as they really are—that is, he begins to form an image such that, acting in terms of that image, he will achieve his goal. It is also evident that perception determines values: as we see things, so we act. But equally the success or failure of our action will determine our later vision. It is evident too that much of the change which in psychotherapy seems to be change in the patient's system of values seems, subjectively to that patient, to be a change in the way he perceives things. Action would seem to be the middle term in which perception and value meet.

4. It is well known that wish and perception partially coincide. Indeed this discovery is one of Freud's greatest contributions. Not only does every human being tend to see in the external world (and in himself) that which he wishes to be the case; but having seen in the external world something even disastrous, he must still wish his information to be true. He must act in terms of what he knows—good or evil—and when he acts he will meet with frustration and pain if things are not as he "knows" them to be. Therefore he must, in a certain sense, wish them to be as he "knows" they are.

5. The preceding paragraph brings up a matter of great theoretical importance: the problem of the relation between the concept "information" and the concept "negative entropy." Wiener (180) has argued that these two concepts are synonymous; and this statement, in the opinion of the writers, marks the greatest single shift in human thinking since the days of Plato and Aristotle, because it unites the natural and social sciences and finally resolves the problems of teleology and the body-mind dichotomy which Occidental thought has inherited from classical Athens. The concept of entropy and the Second Law of Thermodynamics which defines this concept are, however, hazy in the minds of many social scientists, and therefore some explanation is necessary.

(a) According to the Second Law of Thermodynamics, **any**

system of objects in a state from which work can be obtained will tend to change away from this state if random events are allowed to occur. The classic instance is the case of molecules of gas sorted into two containers according to their velocity (i.e., temperature). For such a system, Carnot pointed out, the "available energy" of the system is a function of the difference of temperature between the gas in the two containers. He also pointed out that such available energy—i.e., "negative entropy" —will be diminished either if the system is made to do work or if random events are allowed to occur such as a mixing of the molecules. The system will change toward a more random or probable state—i.e., toward "entropy."

(b) It is evident that Carnot and the engineers generally were applying their own value system as engineers when they enunciated these generalizations. To them "available energy" was a desideratum in the cylinders of heat engines.

(c) The probability law will, however, apply in all cases, and is not restricted to instances in which the sorting is by temperature; or to instances from which physical work can be obtained. If, for example, a pack of cards is in any state which we call "sorted," any shuffling of the pack will probably upset this arrangement.

(d) Wiener points out that the whole range of entropy phenomena is inevitably related to the fact of our knowing or not knowing what state the system is in. If nobody knows how the cards lie in the pack, it is to all intents and purposes a shuffled pack. Indeed, this ignorance is all that can be achieved by shuffling.

(e) From this it follows that the "system" which is really referred to in statements about sorting and negative entropy includes the speaker, whose information and value systems are thus inextricably involved in every such statement which he makes.

6. The relation between information and value becomes still more evident when we consider the asking of questions and other forms of seeking information. We may compare the seeking of information with the seeking of values. In the seeking of values it is clear that what happens is that a man sets out to "trick"

the Second Law of Thermodynamics. He endeavors to interfere with the "natural" or random course of events, so that some otherwise improbable outcome will be achieved. For his break-fast, he achieves an arrangement of bacon and eggs, side by side, upon a plate; and in achieving this improbability he is aided by other men who will sort out the appropriate pigs in some distant market and interfere with the natural juxtaposition of hens and eggs. Similarly in his courtship, he will endeavor to make a particular girl fall in love with him—and prevent her from behaving in a random manner. Briefly, in value seeking he is achieving a coincidence or congruence between something in his head—an idea of what breakfast should be—and something external, an actual arrangement of eggs and bacon. He achieves this coincidence by altering the external objects and events. In contrast, when he is seeking information, he is again trying to achieve a congruence between "something in his head" and the external world; but now he attempts to do this by altering what is in his head.

Negative entropy, value, and information, are in fact alike in so far as the system to which these notions refer is the man plus environment, and in so far as, both in seeking information and in seeking values, the man is trying to establish an otherwise improbable congruence between ideas and events.

7. From what has been said above, it would be natural for the reader to ask a question somewhat as follows: "If the value system and the system of codification of information are really only aspects of the same central phenomenon, then how would you translate statements in terms of the one into statements in terms of the other?" Indeed, only by an adequate answer to this question can we make clear what we here mean by the two "aspects" of the system. We now attempt this:

Whatever communication we consider, be it the transmission of impulses in a neural system or the transmission of words in a conversation, it is evident that every message in transit has two sorts of "meaning" (117), (155). On the one hand, the message is a statement or report about events at a previous moment, and on the other hand it is a command—a cause or stimulus for events at a later moment. Consider the case of three neurons.

A, B, and C, in series, so that the firing of A leads to the firing of B, and the firing of B leads to the firing of C. Even in this extremely simple case, the message transmitted by B has the two sorts of meanings referred to above (105). On the one hand it can be regarded as a "report" to the effect that A fired at a previous moment; and on the other hand it is a "command" or cause for C's later firing. The same thing is true of all verbal communication, and indeed of all communication whatsoever. When A speaks to B, whatever words he uses will have these two aspects: they will tell B about A, conveying information about some perception or knowledge which A has; and they will be a cause or basis for B's later action. In the case of language, however, the presence of these two meanings may be obscured by syntax. A's words may have the syntax of command, which will partly obscure their report aspects. For example, A may say "Halt!" and B may obey the command ignoring the informational aspects—e.g., the fact that A's words indicate some perception or other mental process of which his command is an indication. Or A's words may have the syntax of report, and B may fail to notice that this report has influenced him in a certain direction.

This double aspect of all communication is, of course, a commonplace of the psychiatric interview and is indeed the basis of a large part of all differences between the content of consciousness and the unconscious. The patient is continually aware of only one aspect of what he is saying—whether it be the "report" or the "command"—and the psychiatrist is continually calling his attention to that aspect which he would prefer not to recognize. Conversely, the psychiatrist is not infrequently and often deliberately influencing the patient by comments and interpretations which have the appearance of report but which in fact exert influence upon the patient. Be that as it may, from the point of view of the present study, we state flatly that all communication has this duality of aspect and note that it remains important to investigate which of these aspects is perceived by the selective awareness of therapist and patient respectively in the given context.

Returning now to the question of translating statements

about the codification of information into statements about the value system, it seems that this translation contains exactly the same type of difficulty that would be presented by the task of translating the report aspect of A's message into its command aspect. This difficulty may be summarized in the following form: that the translation is impossible unless we have total knowledge of B's psychological mechanism. If A says that the cat is on the mat, the observer can predict B's responses to this news only in so far as he knows B's psychic habits, especially his evaluation of cats and mats and the inhibitions which may prevent him from acting as he would like to act.

Into the above discussion, a fallacy has been allowed to creep. The question was how to translate statements about A's codification system into statements about A's value system; but for this question has been substituted a different question of predicting what will be the stimulus or command content of A's message as received by B. In the analogy, we have compared the integrated individual who both perceives and acts to a relationship involving two individuals, one (A) who perceives, codifies, and transmits information, and another (B) who acts upon this information. Any such comparison is clearly fallacious. Indeed, it is our thesis that precisely this fallacy is involved in all attempts to distinguish between the value system of an individual and his codification system. All attempts to translate from one system to another will inevitably lead to some fallacy of this order. They lead to describing the individual as though he were two separate persons, a perceiver and an active agent.

Let us therefore now attempt to put the two halves of the individual together. We may say that he perceives, and we may say that he acts as a result of his perception, but these two statements are really inseparable. Our only data about his codification of external events are derived from his reactions (introspective reports being only a special case among other reactions). His reactions are, in fact, a further stage of codification, another complex transformation derived from the original events. Two steps of codification or transformation have occurred between external events and the individual's reaction to these events, and the observer has access only to the "product" (in the mathematical sense) of the two steps when superimposed. From this product it is impossible to arrive at any knowledge of either stage as a separate process. If the individual studied makes evident mistakes in his reaction to external events—as the patient often does—the observer has absolutely no means of knowing wherein the error lies. The subject may have "perceived" the events wrongly, or he may have translated correct perceptions into wrong actions: but which of these errors has occurred the external observer cannot tell. The question is unanswerable and therefore unreal.

8. This, then, would be our conclusion in regard to the nature of the relationship between codification and evaluation—that these two processes may occur separately, but that for the purposes of all scientific discussion they must be treated as a single process and studied through the complex characteristics of the relation between input (i.e., stimulus) and output (i.e., reaction) of the individual.

9. But there is also this point: that, whether or not it is realistic to separate two aspects of the single process, human beings in Occidental cultures do really talk and act as though these processes were separable. Right or wrong, the idea that value and codification are different phenomena modifies behavior and the events of therapy. Human beings in their interaction in therapy and in daily life draw inferences about each other's values and motivations, phrasing these inferences (so far as they phrase them at all) in terms of value and perception —i.e., in terms which presume a division in what, according to the present argument, should be grouped under a single heading of "codification-evaluation." In a later section we shall argue that it is specifically these inferences that are crucial to therapeutic change.

10. Lastly, a word must be said about consciousness, not to solve the ancient problems presented by this strange subjective datum but rather to indicate how those problems are related to the conceptual scheme which is here offered. Whatever may be the mechanistic or spiritual base of the phenomenon, it is certainly a special case of codification and reductive simplification of information about certain parts of the wider psychic life. It is, of course, true that the presence of consciousness de-

notes an extraordinary complication of the psyche, and many specifically human problems and maladjustments arise from this mirroring of a part of the total psyche in the field of consciousness. But still the fact seems clear that the content of consciousness is an extreme reduction, derived from the total rich continuum of psychic events. Every such reduction is a transformation or codification in the same sense in which the terms are here used and, as in all other cases of codification, the nature of the transformation is not itself subject to direct introspection or voluntary control. This, indeed, is the point which we wish to stress: that while the (possibly illusory) sense of free will is closely bound up with the subjective experience of consciousness, the process by which items are selected for focusing in the mirror of consciousness is itself an unconscious process, not, at any given moment, subject to any exercise of the will. Over time, an individual can "train himself" to various sorts of special awareness, and to this extent he can modify the codification of ideas entering consciousness. But at a given instant, the determinism of that instant is seemingly complete.

Many schools of therapy operate upon the premise that therapeutic change is actually a change in the scope and content of consciousness, and the matter is therefore important to the present study. For present purposes, however, the problem of such changes is rephrased as follows: We assume that the person who "trains himself" does so as a result of past experience —especially interpersonal experience—which has determined his ability and motivation to undertake such changes. Such changes occur in therapy, and we must ask therefore about the interpersonal events and contexts of therapy which motivate and facilitate these changes. In brief, the introduction of consciousness as a concept will not profoundly modify the type of question which is here studied.

SELECTIVE AND PROGRESSIONAL INTEGRATION

Certain characteristics of the total codification-evaluation process will now be considered, in such a way as to pose questions about changes in this process—such changes being, according to our hypothesis, essential to therapy.

Broadly, there seem to be two sorts of process within the

general area of codification-evaluation. These may be contrasted by considering two extreme examples. The first process we shall call decision by selective integration, and we shall exemplify it by a man's making a choice among a number of objects. To make this choice, he recognizes the specific objects as apples, oranges, pears, etc., and he knows from past experience which he likes and what actions and gratifications will be involved in eating the various sorts. If there is an unknown fruit among them, this too will be categorized as "unknown," and this category will have positive or negative value, determined by past experience. In this process of selective integration, the man categorizes and evaluates alternatives according to impressions derived from past experience, equating and differentiating elements of the unique present according to his experience with other elements in his unique past.

In contrast, an entirely different process of decision seems to occur in, for example, an extemporizing dancer. For any given movement within a sequence of movements, it is evident that some type of selection occurs which is different from the choice of a fruit of a given species. The dancer's choice is influenced to a much greater extent by the ongoing characteristics of his sequence of action, and even, perhaps, by the ongoing dancing of a partner. This second type of decision we shall call decision by progressional integration, and we shall amplify the example by saying that the phenomenon is not confined to activities involving rapid physical movement, though the movement of the dancer is a convenient model to characterize the state of any person whose actions involve relatively rapid complex movement in "psychological space." It seems that this type of progressional integration is especially characteristic for action sequences in which the component acts are imperfectly differentiated and categorized, and in which speed of decision is important.

Both the selective and progressional processes are probably present in some degree in every human decision. The man who is choosing fruit is in part influenced by the ongoing sequences of his own metabolism, by his preference for certain sequences of taste, and by the intricacies of ongoing courtesy between himself and any other person present. To this extent he acts on a progressional integration. Correspondingly, the dancer may envisage alternatives of action (including the alternative of ceasing to dance), and he may introspectively believe that he is choosing among these categories. In general, it seems that the selective and progressional phenomena may occur each within a frame defined by the other: After he has decided to eat a certain fruit, the details of the act of eating may be progressively determined within the framework of the selective decision. And conversely, in ongoing decisions involving long spans of time it is common for an individual to act selectively at every step and to discover that he has gradually made a major decision (e.g., the choice of a profession) by some progressional process.

It is clear, too, that persons differ in the relative importance of these two processes. Some will try to act selectively in contexts where the time relations of the actions would seem to demand progressional integration; while others will let themselves be guided by a progressional psychological *élan* even in contexts where the alternatives could have been more conventionally evaluated in categories. From a therapeutic point of view, it is important that certain types of patients benefit by learning to categorize the universe, while others must learn to act more freely in terms of progressional integration.

It also seems that cultures differ in the extent to which individuals within a given culture live according to one mode or another; and that cultures may differ in the relationship between these modes. In Balinese culture, for example, where the character structure of the individual seems to be codified in kinesthetic terms and feelings rather than in terms of the zonal modalities (21), it is conspicuous that categories of selective integration are necessary to enable any individual to determine what type of progressional action sequence he should follow. The selective categories of the social organization, in Balinese culture, are the major premises, within the terms of which the individual may behave with a very free progressional integration. He must know the caste of the individual whom he is talking to before he can talk at all. He must know the nature of the context in which he finds himself at the moment, but once these categories are determined, he is free to act in terms of a progressional spontaneity which many Occidentals envy. Occidental cultures seem often to promote a compulsive categorization of the details of behavior, while leaving the individual a greater freedom to act in terms of progressional integration in regard to the wider decisions. These generalizations are, however, liable to be reversed or modified from individual to individual.

DIVERSITIES OF CODIFICATION

As mentioned above, people vary in the degree to which they perceive and act upon their own and other people's words and actions as "reports" or commands. Likewise, people vary in the degree to which they operate selectively or progressionally. The present section follows up these two statements of variation among individuals with an attempt to construct a general scheme, sufficiently abstract to classify the various orders of contrast in codification and evaluation which may conceivably occur among individuals. To enumerate all varieties of human codification and evaluation would be a superhuman task; all that we here attempt is to set up a framework of categories within which the many varieties may be interrelated—a task which should not be beyond the wit of man.

In order to set up such a scheme, it is convenient to start from a non-human model which will be totally incapable of the complex codifications and evaluations which are characteristic of man. We can then build up our notions about man by deliberately and systematically anthropomorphizing the model.

Figure 1 is offered as such a model, and represents the minimum system about which we can meaningfully talk. The arrows represent causal chains, and the entire diagram represents an entity consisting of an internal self-corrective causal circuit which acts upon and is acted upon by an environment. The reader who desires a more concrete picture may imagine, if he pleases, either a protozoan engaged in positive heliotropism or a servomechanism seeking a target. In any case, however the model is embodied, it is certainly incapable of the complex codifications and evaluations which are relevant for this study. At most it may distinguish elements of the environment ("light,"

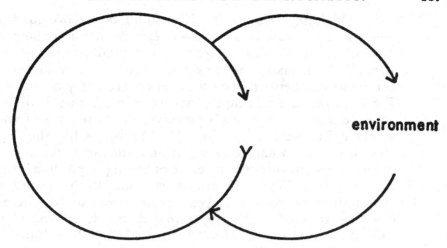

environment

"no light," etc.), but certainly it will not be capable of conceptualizing such notions as "I perceive light," "I seek light," "The perception of light is a pleasure," or "The light compels me to go toward it." In the actions and self-corrections of such simple tropic systems, no evaluative principles of these higher types can be perceived, and it is such principles as these that we seek to classify. The model, then, has this usefulness: it presents us with a *carte blanche* for systematic anthropomorphizing.

We shall later attempt to consider the more complex case of interaction between two such models, exemplifying the possibilities for codification and evaluation of the processes of interaction between persons. Here for heuristic simplicity, we deal first with the organisms vis-à-vis an impersonal environment and mention those types of complexity conceivable in this simple but unreal case.

The following types of codification-evaluation present themselves, and are listed according to a logical order. (We do not suggest that evolution followed this course.)

1. *Discrimination of perceived entities in that arc of the total circuit which we call environment.* We here refer to the recognition of environmental Gestalten of various types and to the classification and delimitation of these ("oak trees," "light,"

etc.). This categorization is trivial so far as our present study is concerned, because it is relatively easy in ongoing communication between persons to iron out misunderstandings at this level, and especially easy to do so when verbal communication can be supplemented by pointing at concrete objects and events. For purposes of mapping the possible diversities of codification, we note that the organism's perceived Gestalten are in all cases arbitrary but interdependent. The organism is, like the scientist, free to delimit whatever systems and entities it pleases in the external world; but certain entities having been discriminated, later discriminations will follow according to the system of discrimination to which the organism is committed by the earlier discriminations. Having discriminated "oak trees" from "light," the discrimination of "elms" from "oaks" and of "blue" from "red" is likely to follow.

2. *Subdivision of that sub-circuit which we call the organism.* Here we refer to the organism's recognition and discrimination of parts of the body, sensations, actions, and the like. With this step it becomes possible to associate sensations with parts of the body, and perhaps to conceptualize purposes in terms of localized sensation—already a conceptual narrowing of the totality of interaction between the organism and the environment. Also, perhaps with this step it becomes possible to falsify parts of the body image and to project such falsification onto other parts of the total circuit, especially onto the environment.

3. *Subdivision of the total circuit into two parts, the self and the environment.* In ontogeny this step is no doubt facilitated by the presence of other similar organisms and by the recognition of these as similar to the self, and it is possible that no concept of the self could be reached in the absence of other similar organisms. But, be that as it may, the differentiation of the self from the environment is conceptually possible without the presence of other organisms and therefore is discussed at this point. Such a differentiation, like all those with which we deal, is in a certain sense arbitrary, and its arbitrary nature is clear when we consider the simplified model from which we started. The imaginary organism is free to draw a closed line anywhere on this diagram and to regard everything inside this

line as "self" while everything on the outside is "environment"; and indeed the usefulness of the model is that it stresses this freedom.

Figure 2 represents the case in which the organism includes

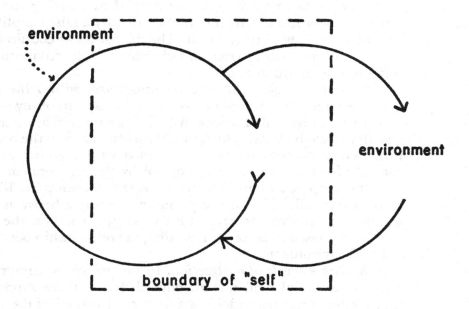

within the self various objects and events outside his skin but intimately connected with him, while he labels as parts of the environment certain of his own body parts or functions of which he is perhaps dimly aware or over which he feels that he has no control. There is, in fact, no right way of delimiting the self; failure to communicate, frustration, and ultimately hostility and pathology may follow if organisms who have conflicting premises on this subject seek to communicate. Further, their communication will be rendered the more difficult inasmuch as neither is likely to be fully aware of what he himself includes in his concept of self. To be able to conceptualize "I include such-and-such in my 'self' " is already a much more complex achievement than the simpler "I am and there are things which are not me."

Recognition of the phenomena of conceptualization will be discussed below.

4. *Conceptualization of control between self and environment.* This again is a step beyond the mere differentiation of self from environment and enables the organism to perceive the environment as coercive or to see himself as coercing the environment—either of which notions is usually a false simplification of the reality of interaction. The diversities of codification will include all those attributions of passivity and activity to the self and the environment.

5. *Conceptualization of separate causal arcs within the self.* Here we refer to such premises as "I am the captain of my soul" and the mind-body dichotomy. All of these are perhaps derivative from a codification, which would identify parts of the organism itself as "environmental," combined with premises about control of the environment or control by the environment. In fact, the supposed internal splitting of the individual is likely to be a symbolic echo of the presumed relations between the self and the environment; or, vice versa, splits within the self may be expressed in premises regarding the relationship between self and environment.

6. *Multiple levels of abstraction.* In the preceding paragraph a step of a special kind was introduced. It was there supposed that the organism may adopt as a device for codifying the relations between causal arcs within the self, certain premises formerly used in the codification of a relationship between the self and the environment. We note in passing that such a proceeding, based on analogy, may well lead to error, but does not of necessity do so. It is, in fact, the possibility and nature of such steps in codification that concern us, rather than their validity. In sum, the organism perceives Gestalt A and Gestalt B and codifies on the assumption that there is a relationship (of likeness or unlikeness) between A and B. This proceeding involves, either explicitly or implicitly, a higher level of abstraction than that involved in the primary codification of the two Gestalten. The "likeness" or "unlikeness" is more abstract than either Gestalt A or Gestalt B. By steps of this kind the codification system of the organism becomes more and more elaborate

and may contain many levels of abstraction, the interrelations of which are capable of great diversity.

7. *Gestalten involving time spans of varying lengths.* The organism may see a single movement as an "act" or may see whole sequences of events, including both his own actions and results of that action as having a unity or purpose or failure. He may even conceptualize the limitations of his own life and with such notions, symbolically extended, he may see an initiation ceremony or even his own therapeutic experience as a sort of death and rebirth.

8. *The reification of concepts.* Finally the organism may turn upon its own codification system in various ways. As soon as sufficient complexity is reached to permit of two or more levels of abstraction, the organism becomes able to treat abstractions of a higher level as though they were equivalent to abstractions of a lower level. In brief, the organism may reify any concept within the wide scope already indicated above, and may endow this concept with, for example, causal or controlling efficacy. "Morality" (an abstraction derived from the actions and the words of the self and others) may be seen as "binding" upon actions of the self; the organism may respect or may revolt against "cultural conventions"; he may even sneer at or repudiate "death" (an abstraction about which he can, in the nature of the case, have no subjective knowledge).

This very brief survey of the orders of complexity and possible diversity in codification will serve to prepare the reader for the generalization that it is possible for the organism to commit many types of error in its codification and interpretation of the world. The next section will attempt to define some of these types of error.

INTERNAL CONTRADICTIONS OF CODIFICATION-EVALUATION

The previous section discusses the conceivable scope of variation in codification-evaluation but stops short of considering the discrepancies which may occur within such systems. The present section adds a new level of complexity by asserting that, conceivably, contradiction (i.e., ambivalence) may occur in any of the types of codification there outlined; that such internal contradictions may occur at any level of abstraction; and that a given contradiction may in fact involve two or more such levels.

In daily life and psychiatric experience, it is common to observe that a person may see and evaluate similar events in one way in one set of circumstances and in quite a different way in another set of circumstances; and the contrast of circumstances which determines such a change may be either internal (for example, a shift of mood) or external (that which is approved and valued in war may be regarded with horror in time of peace). Trouble arises the moment the individual fails to make due allowance for the contexts of his evaluation and equates, for example, certain actions which are appropriate in war with certain similar actions in peacetime. He thus creates for himself a concept or Gestalt (e.g., "violence") which is charged with both positive and negative value.

Perhaps if human beings were capable of maintaining clarity about the contexts of perception and evaluation, they might avoid the complex internal and interpersonal conflicts which result from such contradictions. But this they cannot achieve. If it were possible never to confuse a given type of event (E^1) in one set of internal or external circumstances (C^1) with similar events (E^2) in other sets of circumstances (C^2, etc.), all would be well. But this is impossible, short of sacrificing the whole of Gestalt codification. The price which man pays for the economy which Gestalt codification permits is his proneness to ambivalence. After all, the great economy which this type of codification permits is due precisely to the fact that it permits us to identify E^1 with E^2 (e.g., to recognize a square as a square though it is presented in many different ways). Codification in terms of Gestalten permits us to summarize experience, and it is this summarization of experience that results in ambivalence.

Further, a second sort of internal discrepancy in the codification-evaluation system follows from the fact that every summary is an arbitrary condensation of the unsummarized data. Every Gestalt label is a man-made categorization of events in a universe which might be categorized in infinitely various ways. Even in the instant of perception or action, the individual is applying many such labels to the given set of events or objects. Inevitably there will be cases in which such overlapping labels will have contrary value or contrary implications for action. With such a variety of possibilities for internal discrepancy, it is perhaps hopeless to attempt any complete survey of the possibilities for

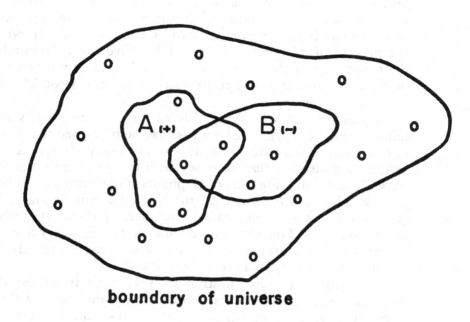

boundary of universe

ambivalence. However, since certain types can be defined with some rigor, these will be listed:

(a) Cases of overlapping Gestalt labeling in which the Gestalten are of the same level of abstraction. These cases may be described in a diagram. Figure 3 represents a universe of objects and events as perceived by an individual, including the individual's own actions among these. Within this universe, he perceives a sub-set of items as together making a Gestalt unity, A; he also perceives another sub-set which make up another Gestalt unity, B. Now, if there are items in common between A and B, and if A is positively valued and B negatively valued, the result will be a form of ambivalence. The items in the area of overlap will be positively valued when they are perceived as parts of A, but negatively valued when they are perceived as parts of B.

In this type of contradiction, it is important to note that there is no necessary tendency for the perception of the Gestalt A to promote perception of the Gestalt B and vice versa; rather, we would expect the perception of the one to hinder the perception of the other. It is, however, easy to imagine instances in which the perception of either Gestalt might drive the individual to the perception of the other. These would be cases intermediate between the first types of contradiction and the second, which we now describe.

(b) Cases which are comparable in form to the famous Russellian paradox (177). The paradox may be presented as follows: A man classifies entities into classes, and every class which he defines establishes a class of other entities which are non-members. He notes that the class of elephants is itself not an elephant but that the class of not-elephants is itself a not-elephant. He generalizes that some classes are members of themselves while others are not. Thereby, he establishes two larger classes of classes. He then must decide: is the class of classes which are not members of themselves a member of itself?

If the answer to this question is "yes," then it follows that this class must be one of those which are not members of themselves, since all the members are of this type—and therefore the answer must really be "no." If on the other hand the answer is "no," then the class must be a member of that other class whose characteristic it is that its members are members of themselves —so the answer must be "yes"; and so on. If the answer is "yes" then it must be "no"—but if it is "no" then it must be "yes."

Another paradox with essentially the same structure is that presented by a man who says, "I am lying." Is he telling the truth?

A mechanical model of such an oscillating or paradoxical system may be of use to the reader. Such a model is the ordinary electric buzzer or house bell. This machine consists of an electromagnet acting upon an armature (a light metal spring) through which the current which activates the magnet must pass. The armature is so placed that the circuit is broken whenever the magnet is active and causes the spring to bend. But the current is re-established by the relaxation of the spring when the magnet ceases to act. We may translate this system into logical propositions by labeling that position of the spring which closes the circuit as "yes"; and labeling the contrasting position which breaks the circuit as "no." The following pair of propositions can then be stated:

1. If the spring is in "yes," the circuit is closed and the electromagnet operates; therefore the spring must go to "no."

2. But if the spring is in "no," the magnet is not operating, and the spring must therefore go to "yes."

Thus the implications of "yes" involve "no"; and the implications of "no" involve "yes." The model illustrates precisely the Russellian paradox, inasmuch as the "yes" and "no" are each of them being applied at two levels of abstraction. In Proposition 1, "yes" refers to position, while "no" refers to direction of change; in proposition 2, "no" refers to position, while "yes" refers to direction of change. The "no" to which "yes" is an answer is therefore not the same as the "no" which is an answer to "yes."

Similarly the paradox presented by the statement "I am lying" can be traced to a confusion of levels of abstraction. The three words which are all we have to go on are simultaneously both a statement (level 1) and a statement (level 2) about the falsity of this first statement; and the second statement is of a higher order of abstraction than the first. In Russell's formal presentation of the paradox in terms of "classes of classes" the levels of abstraction are made explicit and the paradox is ruled out of order.

This matter of the paradoxes is here discussed at some length because it is impossible to go far in thinking about communication and codification without running into tangles of this type and because similar tangles of levels of abstraction are common in the premises of human culture (Chapter 8) and in psychiatric patients. In fact, this is the type of internal contradiction which Korzybski (90) and the school of general semantics attempt to correct in their therapy. Their treatment consists in training the patient not to confuse his levels of abstraction. In fact, their treatment follows the lines of Russell's resolution of the paradox, which he attempted by asserting the rule that no class shall ever be regarded as a member of itself—because to do so would be to confuse levels of abstraction.

The reader, if he submits himself to the experience of thinking through the Russellian paradox, will observe that a time element is involved. For a moment it is satisfactory to accept the answer "yes," but he will observe that as he perceives the more intimate details of the Gestalt set up by this answer, he is driven to reject it. Then for a moment the answer "no" is acceptable until its implications are perceived—and so on. From the psychological point of view, this time characteristic is important: the phenomenon is not one of static indecision, but one of "oscillation" in time. Probably everybody has had the experience of similar sequences in real life in which increasing familiarity with a Gestalt leads to its rejection in favor of some other which in turn later becomes unacceptable. These, in fact, are systems of contradiction in which temporary acceptance of one pole promotes preference for the other and vice versa. The attempt to resolve the conflict in favor of one of its polarities *ipso facto* generates a preference for the contrasting pole. This mechanism is therefore very different from that discussed in (a) above, though the two mechanisms may conceivably work in combination.

(c) A third form of apparent internal contradiction in the codification-evaluation system is that of circular preference (106). When possibilities are offered in pairs, it may happen that A is preferred to B; and B is preferred to C; and C is preferred to A. In such a system, there will presumably be impossibility of decision when the three possibilities are simultaneously present. The data upon preference systems of this kind are meager, but the phenomenon is of great theoretical importance. The phenomenon is said to occur in experiments with aesthetic preference—e.g., when rectangles are presented in pairs, and the subject is asked to express preference for one member of each pair.

The mechanisms involved in circular preference may be various: (a) It may be that in the Gestalt "A plus B" the evaluation of each member is a function of the presence of the other; so that when B is presented in the presence of C, and the Gestalt "B plus C" is seen, B will be evaluated differently and perhaps according to different criteria. (b) The mechanism of decision may consist of multiple linked sub-entities each with its own preference. The total mechanism of decision would then be something like a voting population; and notoriously in such systems, if there are three voters (or three equal parties) it is possible for that voter who sends no candidate to the election to swing the decision to that one of the other two candidates whom he prefers. (c) McCulloch has outlined a possible type of neurological circuit which will produce a similar result, and a related phenomenon obtains among the alternative solutions to certain types of Von Neumannian games (168).

Whether there are other types of internal contradiction or whether all are ultimately reducible to the three types mentioned above, is unknown.

ONE-WAY COMMUNICATION: THE UNOBSERVED OBSERVER

Before considering the more complex case of two or more organisms in mutual communication, it is worth while to ask how an observer, of whom the single observed organism is unaware, might build up inferences about that organism's system of codification-evaluation. This case, of involuntary one-way communication, will provide an important generalization relevant to more complex cases.

If, for example, the observer sees the organism moving in a straight line toward some target such as a source of light, he will not with this limited observation be able even to recognize a tropism. Repeated observations of the same type will still not help him, except to verify a very broad hypothesis that the coincidence between the direction of motion of the organism and the direction in which the light is located is due to something more than chance. He will not know that the direction of motion is selected by any process within the organism. To learn more, either the observer must perform repeated experiments, or he must observe repeatedly that the organism corrects itself every time the course deviates from the direction of the target. Moreover, the observer's experiments will necessarily take the form of placing the organism in error (e.g., he will place the light somewhere not in the direction in which the organism is traveling and will then look to see what the organism will do). And from this it follows that the data which the observer obtains by experiment are of the same general type as those which he would obtain by observing the organism's self-correction in a variety of circumstances.

From these arguments, the major conclusion follows: That the correction of mistakes is a basic means of communication and is actually the only sort of communication which will permit an unobserved observer to form inferences about the codification-evaluation system of the observed.

The special case in which an organism while performing some action talks to itself and is overheard by an observer is interesting but does not invalidate the above argument: (a) If the observer is unfamiliar with the language of the observed, his only way of reaching an understanding will be by regarding the verbal behavior and the action sequences of the observed as a single system of ongoing self-correction. In this way he will finally discover what the words mean, and each utterance will be meaningful as selected by the observed in a process of self-correction. The observer will learn, in fact, the polarities of codification in the language; he will be able to assign to each word positive meaning, in so far as the word delimits a set of negated alternatives. (b) If the observer already partly or fully knows the language of the observed, he will tend to operate by identifying himself with the latter, ascribing to the observed his own understanding of the words used. In doing this he will either learn nothing new about the latter's codification system, or he will discover that he himself is making mistakes in interpreting what is said; as regards these parts of the codification-evaluation system of the observed, he will be, in fact, in the position of not knowing the language. In any case, unless the verbal stream is accompanied by action and is self-corrective in regard to the action, the observer will be able to learn nothing about the language.

This generalization echoes what has been said earlier as to the nature of codification-evaluation. It was there stated that in both codification and evaluation the universe is structured into a network. In the case of codification, the network is one whose nodes are the bi-polar or multi-polar discriminations of perception. In the case of evaluation, the network has nodes which define the polarities of preference. In studying the mistakes and self-corrections of the organism, the observer is in fact getting the data necessary to map out the polarities of these networks. He will learn—albeit laboriously—what discriminations the organism can make, upon what cues it acts, whether it is able to perceive any characteristics of its own actions, how the action system is related to cues given, and so on.

INTRAPERSONAL COMMUNICATION: THE SELF-OBSERVER

A question of very great practical and theoretical importance in the psychiatric world concerns the limitations of self-observation and self-therapy. A corresponding question strikes anthropologists, who are well aware that it is especially difficult for a student to obtain insight into his own culture. It is orthodox among anthropologists today to believe that deep and articulate insight into one's own culture can only be obtained through the comparative method. Be that as it may, it is certain that awareness of his own cultural premises has come to man late in his history and has been aided by comparison between cultures. It is natural to draw an analogy between anthropology and psychiatry in this matter, and to suggest that the need for a comparative approach in anthropology is comparable to the need, in therapy, for another human being (the therapist) different from the self, against whom as a background the peculiarities of the self can be seen. The analogy cannot, however, be pushed too far. It is curious that while the especially important item in an anthropologist's training is his first-hand experience of a completely foreign culture, the corresponding item in the training of a psychiatrist is his own psychoanalysis.

Opinions differ as to what an individual can do in the way of obtaining insight into his own personality unaided by any therapist, and the problem is complicated by the evident fact that therapeutic progress may, under certain circumstances, occur without insight. It is possible that a therapist is necessary if the patient is to achieve insight but that other types of progress can occur without his presence.

In the present study the problems of self-observation are

relevant as part of the base from which we go on to inquire into interpersonal communication. Briefly, the question is: What are the limitations of self-observation as a process by which an individual may obtain new understanding or information about his own codification-evaluation system?

The problem has many branches: (a) It would be desirable to describe the phenomena of self-observation in some way which will not personify a self within the self. (b) The question calls for a definition of what is meant by "new" understanding as distinct from a working out of pre-existing contradictions within the individual's codification-evaluation system. (c) A formal examination is necessary of the actual limits upon self-discovery which arise from the fact that an individual can—of necessity—perceive his own life and actions only in terms of his own system of codification-evaluation. He is, in all cases, unable to perceive the characteristics of the system in terms of which he perceives.

Of these problems it is the third that is of special interest to the present study. The epistemological problem of consciousness and the nature of the self within the self we propose to postpone as being for the present beyond the reach of scientific examination. It has, indeed, been suggested that the subjective experience of consciousness is determined by internal conflict or contradiction. Such a hypothesis would partly remove the problem of consciousness from the epistemological field and place it in the area of the second question proposed above—that of the working out of pre-existing internal contradictions. This second question, in turn, may be postponed in favor of the third, which has the heuristic advantage of greater simplicity. If we can set limits to the possibility of self-perception in an organism not made complex by internal contradiction, these limits will be relevant for any consideration of the more complex cases.

We now consider the possibilities of self-perception in the unconflicted organism. Again, for heuristic reasons, we consider first the case of an organism in an environment such that the premises of codification-evaluation within the organism are true and sufficient for that environment in which it lives. Such a hypothetical organism will always achieve its goals by means of those sorts of codification and self-correction which are characteristic for the organism, and it will not strive after any impossible goals. The question is whether, from such a sequence of automatic successes, the organism can ever achieve a new insight into its own automatic processes of self-correction.

The answer is surely a flat negative. From all that is known about learning, it would follow that in such a hypothetical case, not only no new insight but even no learning of any kind will occur. Indeed, the hypothetical case here discussed is precisely that of the abstract "player" in a Von Neumannian game.

If, on the other hand, there are contradictions, not within the organism but between the premises of the organism and those which obtain in the environment, then the position is entirely different. We know, as a fact of behavioristic experiment, that in such cases an organism which formerly appeared to act in terms of one premise system may after a period of trial and error gradually or suddenly begin to act as though in terms of another and better-adapted system. Further, we know from introspective reports that such learning may be accompanied by a change in the organism's conscious perception of the environment.

This again is a problem of mistakes and the correction of mistakes, such as was discussed in the previous section. The organism has been "put in the wrong" by the environment, and now the question is what orders of new information the organism can achieve as a result of going through the whole experience of frustration and self-correction, and achieving that new system of codification and evaluation by which the frustration is reduced. Having been put in the wrong, the organism corrects itself, not merely modifying its action but modifying—more or less profoundly—the basic processes and mechanisms by which actions are related to environmental cues. The "mistake" corrected in this sequence is of a very different order from the act of self-correction which characterized the organism at the outset of the experiment. The organism has now modified its system of self-correction.

The following considerations are relevant to the comparison

between the therapeutic process and such modification of system
as can be achieved by the isolated organism:

1. The change in the isolated organism, in so far as it is
an improvement in adaptation, may be regarded as "therapeutic."

2. It is known from experiment that failure on the part of
the organism to adjust its premises to the conditions of the
environment may be anti-therapeutic and may lead to experimental neurosis. That is, the organism may be affected by the
fact of failure—may, in this sense, have information about
failure.

3. It is unlikely that the old premises will be totally obliter-
ated in the course of the change. Rather, they are likely to survive in modified or "repressed" form. It is possible, in fact, that
the organism at some stage of the process of learning—and perhaps forever afterwards—will entertain conflicting premises with
all the complications which this may entail.

4. It is possible that the organism may achieve new insight
into the environment but very doubtful that it will obtain
new insight into the self. There may be a deutero-learning—
i.e., a learning to learn, or learning about learning (cf. Chapter
8)—such that the organism when again put in the wrong will
be, for example, less anxious because of an acquired faith in
its own ability to deal with such misfortune. But this is only
doubtfully an increased insight into the self. Indeed, it is very
doubtful if such an increase can possibly occur as a result of
the changes which are here considered.

Before the experiment, the organism perceived its own actions
in a certain way determined by the then existing premises; after
the experiment it will perceive itself and its actions in terms
of the new premises. But this is not a change in the order of
self-perception such that we would call it insight. The next
step—to see the self as an entity which has characteristically
accomplished this change—need not occur. A change in the
premises of codification-evaluation need not denote any greater
insight into these premises unless the individual can see this
change as a contrast, comparing himself with what he formerly
was. In such a comparison he is essentially operating as two

persons between whom a contrast can be stated and a comparative method applied leading to greater insight. He is doing something comparable to what normally occurs in a two-person system.

It appears, then, that a two-person system of some sort will always be necessary for insight therapy, but perhaps not for other types of learning. We must, however, also expect that these other types of learning, often themselves therapeutic, will occur in the two-person situation even though the presence of the second person may not be necessary.

The background is now sufficient for the consideration of two-person systems.

COMMUNICATION BETWEEN TWO PERSONS AND METACOMMUNICATION

The next step is to extend what has been said in the previous sections to the phenomena of relationship between two or more persons—anthropomorphic organisms. The primary problem of such communication has been aptly put by Janet Baker (age 10) as follows: "When people thought of a language, how did they think of it if there were no words to think with? After they had thought of it, how did they get other people to understand it? If they went from door to door explaining it, people would think that they had gone crazy because they wouldn't know what the words meant. After the first language was started how were others formed? These are the questions that make me say, 'I wonder how people learned to talk' " (10).

This statement of the matter presents an ultimate problem to which the present inquiry leads; but it must be remembered that between whole human beings, after infancy, there can never be a total lack of mutual understanding. To be sure, there may be misunderstandings, and these may be so profound and dramatic as to seem total, but actually for even misunderstanding to occur, there must be some shared premises of codification-evaluation. Each person must at least have some notions about himself and the other; he must, for example, think of both as alike in being alive and capable of emitting and receiving communication. Indeed, if misunderstanding leads to hostility, it is immediately clear that there must exist common premises regarding anger and pain. The beginnings of a common codification system are latent in our biological nature, our common anatomy and common experience of bodily functioning and maturation. When two human beings meet, they inevitably share many premises about such matters as limbs, sense organs, hunger, and pain.

As regards external cues, there is considerable evidence that among birds, amphibia, fishes, and invertebrates, the members of a species may share an innate tendency to respond in a complex way to a particular sharply defined cue or sequence of cues —a smell, a shape, a size, a patch of color, and the like—originating in other individuals. Such mutual responsiveness may take on the appearance of ongoing interaction. For example, among the sticklebacks there is such an exchange of behaviors between the sexes leading to reproduction. Each sex has a series of specific differentiated responses, and these are interchanged, each partner's response being a stimulus for a new response on the part of the other until finally the male inseminates and stays with the eggs laid by the female in the nest which he has built (164).

In the case of mammals, and especially man, it seems that such innate tendencies to respond in a complex differentiated manner to highly specific external cues are either poorly developed or are changed and blurred by later learning. Man's instinctual equipment is overlaid by cultural elaborations, but there still remain, common to the species, a number of tendencies to respond in a gross or diffuse manner to certain gross or diffuse stimuli, such as loud sounds, removal of support, heat or cold, pain, and the like.

Further, all human beings, as we know the species today, share the notion that language and gesture are media of communication [2] even though every culture has its specific variants

---

[2] The late Doctor Stutterheim, Government Archeologist in Java, used to tell the following story: Somewhat before the advent of the white man, there was a storm on the Javanese coast in the neighborhood of one of the capitals. After the storm the people went down to the beach and found, washed up by the waves and almost dead, a large white monkey of unknown species. The religious experts explained that this monkey had been a member of the court of Beroena,

of these media (184). Even within the culture, the poet may have extraordinarily different premises about the use of language from those held by the advertising man. A dancer may have one set of notions about communicative uses of posture, while the catatonic has another; and yet both share the notion that posture is communicative and, at some more abstract level, both systems of communication probably meet in many common premises about the body. If the contrasting persons live in the same culture, they will also share some vague—even distorted—recognition of the points in which they differ.

In this study, we are specifically concerned with communications between persons who have a large measure of common vocabulary and common setting in the American cultural scene, persons who have lived a great part of their lives in the American variant of Occidental culture. And yet, as between patient and therapist there may be a deep gulf of difference in their premises regarding such matters as were discussed earlier. They may have sharply differing notions as to the boundaries of the self, and each may see his own relationship to other human beings in his own idiosyncratic terms. The paranoiac may believe that the environment is all-powerful and set upon his undoing, but it is impossible to predict what phrasing the therapist may entertain as to his own relationship to his environment. Some therapists are willing and others unwilling to see themselves as shaping their human vis-à-vis. The thesis of this book is that only by communication can therapy occur, and communication will depend upon those premises which the two persons have in common and upon the complexities of the two-person system.

Certain special characteristics emerge in the interpersonal

---

the God of the Sea, and that for some offense the monkey had been cast out by the god whose anger was expressed in the storm. The Rajah gave orders that the white monkey from the sea should be kept alive, chained to a certain stone. This was done. Doctor Stutterheim told me that he had seen the stone and that, roughly scratched on it in Latin, Dutch, and English were the name of a man and a statement of his shipwreck. Apparently this trilingual sailor never established verbal communication with his captors. He was surely unaware of the premises in their minds which labeled him as a white monkey and therefore not a potential recipient of verbal messages: it probably never occurred to him that they could doubt his humanity. He may have doubted theirs.

system which were not significantly present in the hypothetical system containing only one organism:

First, each organism is in receipt of cues having a different order of complexity from those emitted by inanimate objects. Indeed, the messages externally exchanged between organisms must be compared with the intra-organismic processes of codification and evaluation rather than with the data which the organism collects from the inanimate environment. The extraordinary complexity of intra-organismic codification was discussed above, and it was then noted that this complexity is, so far as we know, achieved by very simple neural signals traveling in exceedingly complex pathways, in a network with many billions of synaptic nodes. With the aid of this neural network and possibly other parts of the body, the organism achieves the complex units of internal communication which we call Gestalten. The significant fact, for our present purposes, is that in interpersonal communication, the units and aggregate messages reach this same level because words and postures already refer to complex Gestalten corresponding to some of those which the internal system uses. Communication between persons is of course pathetically impoverished compared with the richness of the intrapersonal consciousness, which in its turn is but an impoverished and restricted version of the total psychic life of the person. But still it is important that the external communications are a codification of the internal psychic life and that the recipient of such communication is receiving an already elaborated product from the psychic life of another individual. In this, interpersonal communication differs profoundly from all perception of the inanimate environment. The perceiving individual must synthesize his data about the inanimate environment into appropriate units and has a certain freedom to do this in an idiosyncratic manner, whereas in receiving a verbal or other personal communication he has less freedom because the matter of the message is already synthesized into Gestalten (words and phrases) by the communicator. Even the recipient's understanding of the message is conditional upon his having become habituated to the narrowly confined conventions of codification which culture imposes.

Each individual receives, of course, sense data of the ordinary kind in regard to the other; each sees and hears the other as a physical entity. But in addition each receives verbal and other symbolic matter from the other, and each has therefore the opportunity to combine these two types of data into a single more complex stream, enriching the verbal flow with simultaneous observations of bodily movement and the like. It was suggested above that in intrapersonal processes the body might serve an analogic function supplementary to the more digital processes of neural thought. We now note that the bodily processes of the other person—his postures, tension, flushing, and the like—serve a corresponding function in interpersonal communication. Each person is able to get a multidimensional view of his vis-à-vis,. enriching the stream of merely verbal symbols with a recognition of bodily processes in the other, and these are more or less intelligible because of common biological background and cultural conditioning.

In illustration, it is worth mentioning a curious detail in which the strictly Freudian analytic session differs from the majority of two-person systems. When the patient is on the couch and the analyst sits on a chair beyond the patient's head, the analyst gets a fair but perhaps sufficient view of the postures and facial expressions of the patient; but the latter is cut off from seeing his therapist. The asymmetries which this arrangement introduces into the therapeutic situation are undoubtedly very complex and surely vary from therapist to therapist and from patient to patient. From the point of view of the present discussion, it is significant that the patient receives only verbal messages from the analyst and so has maximum freedom to build up a fantasy picture of the affective aspects of the analyst's personality. This picture may be later examined when the transference is analyzed. At first the patient, according to his lifetime habit, attempts to make inferences about the analyst in order to tailor his words to fit that person. Later he discovers, perhaps, that in the therapeutic session such tailoring is difficult and he is then thrown back upon speaking and acting as "himself" with minimal aid from such introjected images.

A further characteristic which emerges in the interpersonal

system but which was almost negligible in the simple relation between organism and environment is the real existence of the group as a determinant of the actions and communications of the separate persons. The relation between organism and environment is already an interaction, and in such dynamic systems as a man driving an automobile or a man walking or dancing, the reality of the interactive whole as a determinant of the functions of the constituent parts is clearly recognizable; but when we deal with two-person systems a new sort of integration occurs. The condition for the existence of a determinative group in this sense seems to be that each participant be aware of the perceptions of the other. If I know that the other person perceives me and he knows that I perceive him, this mutual awareness becomes a part determinant of all our action and interaction. The moment such awareness is established, he and I constitute a determinative group, and the characteristics of ongoing process in this larger entity control both individuals in some degree. Here again the shared cultural premises will become effective.

About the evolution of the "group" in this sense, there is little information, but the question of such evolutionary history is worth considering, if only to stress that the group, as defined in terms of mutual awareness of perception, is something different from groups determined merely by mutual irritability or responsiveness. In the case of the sticklebacks (164) mentioned above, there is a complex mutual responsiveness but no evidence which would indicate that either individual is aware of the other's perception. Similarly in the elaborate communication which von Frisch has demonstrated among the bees, there is no reason to believe that such awareness occurs. Probably this evolutionary step occurred for the first time among mammals, and perhaps the phenomenon occurs only among primates and among animals intimately domesticated by man. The matter needs critical investigation.

Operationally, to determine whether a group is of this higher order, it would be necessary at least to observe whether each participant modifies his emission of signals in a self-corrective manner according to his knowledge of whether the signals are likely to be audible, visible, or intelligible to the other participants. Among animals, such self-correction is certainly unusual. Among men it is desirable but not always present.

It would also be important to identify among animals any signals of the following types: (a) signals whose only meaning would be the acknowledgment of a signal emitted by another; (b) signals asking for a signal to be repeated; (c) signals indicating failure to receive a signal; (d) signals which punctuate the stream of signals; and so on. With complete awareness of the other's perception an individual should stop repeating a signal after it has been received and acknowledged by the other individual, and this type of self-correction would indicate mutual perceptive awareness. Correspondingly the lack of such adaptation—often observable in people—would denote imperfect awareness of the other's perception except in those cases where some change in meaning or intensity is conveyed by the repetition of the message. Lastly, the motivation for deliberate falsehood can hardly exist without awareness of the other individual's perception, nor is the falsehood likely to be successful. Thus the occurrence of falsehood becomes an evidence that the group is one based upon mutual awareness of perception.[8]

All these criteria for the existence of mutual awareness build together to give a picture of the entirely new order of communication which emerges with this awareness. For this new order of communication, the term "metacommunication" is here introduced and defined as "communication about communication." We shall describe as "metacommunication" all exchanged cues and propositions about (a) codification and (b) relationship between the communicators. We shall assume that a majority of propositions about codification are also implicit or explicit propositions about relationship and vice versa, so that no sharp line can be drawn between these two sorts of metacommunication. Moreover, we shall expect to find that the qualities and characteristics of metacommunication between persons will de-

[8] The falsehoods implicit in animal mimicry, protective coloration, and the like, present a special problem. Here, according to orthodox hypotheses, the self-corrective system is not the individual animal but the larger system of the total ecology within which natural selection operates correctively upon the population.

pend upon the qualities and degree of their mutual awareness of each other's perception.

If we can recognize the existence of such awareness by observing the individual's self-correction of the signals which he emits (and all the criteria are really only special cases of this self-correction), it follows that a variety of characteristics attributed to the other individual have become relevant in shaping and motivating the behavior of the signaler. The signals are being tailored to fit the signaler's ideas about the receiver. From this point onward the evolution of a number of human habits and characteristics—introjection, identification, projection, and empathy—understandably follows. It even becomes possible for one human individual to coerce another in terms of a correct or incorrect understanding of that other's view of the universe.

This discussion of the importance of interpersonal inference introduces a series of other variables significant for the two-person system which did not appear in hypothetical systems involving only one person. When the system consists of two persons, it is possible for these persons to be either similar or dissimilar in their codification characteristics. They may be alike in the way they perceive the universe and act upon their perception; or they may be different in these respects. The new variable which we note is then the statement of similarity or dissimilarity between the two persons.

Another and different variable which emerges only when two persons communicate will state whether or not the premises of the two persons conflict. It is evidently possible that, though two persons are much alike, the very points in which they resemble each other may be a cause of mutual conflict. If, for example, they are alike in their expansionist goals, these goals may well coincide, and rivalry or jealousy may develop. Indeed, as is well known to educators, the establishment of a competitive relationship between persons is one of the most effective methods of training the participants to a similarity or conformity in their perception and evaluation of the common universe in which they live. More formally stated, these are cases in which A's phrasing of the relationship between A's self and part of the environment is superficially the same as B's phrasing of the relationship between the same part of the environment and B's self. Both may say, "It's mine." Such phrasings are really discrepant, because the two selves do not coincide.

Conversely, when the two persons have evidently different phrasings of the universe, there need not necessarily be conflict. It is possible for the phrasings to be complementary, so that a "fit" occurs (149), and the two individuals may be able to cooperate in an asymmetrical relationship. This occurs, for example, in successful relations between persons of opposite sex. And notably, in such cases it is even not necessary for the persons to understand each other's universe, though it may be important that they recognize the fact of difference. Beyond this recognition, the efforts to understand may result in failure to communicate. These, however, are questions which can hardly be considered apart from the role of the cultural matrix, which will be examined in the next chapter.

8 · CONVENTIONS OF COMMUNICA-TION: Where Validity Depends upon Belief

By Gregory Bateson

IN THE preceding chapter a theory of communication was built up starting from irritability and adaptive action at the very simplest level, and advancing through the phenomena of codification up to the phenomena of mutual awareness of perception. With this last element the theory begins to describe human relations.

In the present chapter what we have to do is to push on into more human matters. Instead of talking about sticklebacks and abstract entities we begin to talk about beings which, schematically at least, resemble people. The particular step towards humanity which we take in this chapter is to examine the idea that *man lives by those propositions whose validity is a function of his belief in them.*

Two sorts of propositions of this kind were mentioned in the preceding chapter. First, the propositions about codification. Such a statement as "The word 'cat' stands for a certain small mammal" is not either true or false. Its truth depends upon agreement between the speakers that it be true. In terms of such agreement they understand each other; or where disagreement occurs they will meet with misunderstanding. And this statement about the word "cat" is only one of a vast category of statements about codification, which category ranges all the way from the conventions of local phonetics up through the conventions of vocabulary to the conventions of syntax; and the same category will include the conventions of timing, pitch, emphasis, tone of voice, and all the other modalities of verbal and nonverbal communication, since all communication involves codification and these are the conventions of codification.

In addition, the preceding chapter contained statements about metacommunication; and this category of statements is a larger genus within which the statements about codification are to be included as a subcategory. When A communicates with B, the mere act of communicating can carry the implicit statement "we are communicating." In fact, this may be the most important message that is sent and received. The wisecracks of American adolescents and the smoother but no less stylized conversations of adults are only occasionally concerned with the giving and receiving of objective information; mostly, the conversations of leisure hours exist because people need to know that they are in touch with one another. They may ask questions which superficially seem to be about matters of impersonal fact —"Will it rain?" "What is in today's war news?"—but the speaker's interest is focused on the fact of communication with another human being. With comparative strangers, we "make conversation" rather than accept the message which would be implicit in silence—the message, "We are *not* communicating." It seems that this message would provoke anxiety because it implies rejection; perhaps also because the message itself is explosive with paradox. If two persons exchange this message, are they communicating?

Many sorts of games are of interest in this connection. An implicit message which is exchanged at bridge tables and on tennis courts is the affirmed agreement between the players as to the rules and goals. By participating in the game, they affirm the fact of communication, and by competing, they affirm the fact of shared value premises.

Similarly, every courtesy term between persons, every inflection of voice denoting respect or contempt, condescension or dependency, is a statement about the relationship between the two persons. Such messages are carried on the stream of verbal communication, and all these messages and their codification determine such matters as role and status, whose truth and stability depend upon implicit or explicit agreement between the persons that the relationship is as indicated. Moreover, all cues which define status and role are metacommunicative, since the recipient of any message is guided in his interpretation of that message and in his resulting action by his view of the relative roles and status between himself and the speaker.

It appears, then, that within the larger genus of metacommunicative propositions, it is possible to recognize at least two subcategories—the propositions about codification and the propositions about interpersonal relationship. It is certain, however, that overlapping frequently occurs between these subcategories and that a very small shift in emphasis or interpretation will cause a given proposition to appear to shift from one subcategory to the other. This shifting character is due to two circumstances: (a) that statements about relationship must still be codified; and (b), that every statement in a given codification is an implicit affirmation of this codification and is therefore in some degree metacommunicative. (When I say, "I see the cat," I am implicitly affirming the proposition that the word "cat" stands for that which I see.) The shifting relation between the propositions of codification and the propositions of human relationship can be illustrated by the following example: The statement "A policeman carries a nightstick as a badge of authority" contains both the statement of status and the statement of how this status is codified; the same example will serve to emphasize that all interpersonal actions are, in some degree, messages. When the policeman uses his nightstick, he is asserting his status in a particular relationship to a particular offender.

The purpose of the present chapter is to examine this whole matter of propositions and implicit premises whose validity depends upon belief.

First, it is necessary to survey, briefly, the occurrence of premises of this order in human life. Broadly, it will be argued that propositions and premises of this kind are scattered through the whole range of life. They are implicit in the phenomena of learning, they recur in the phenomena of character formation, and finally they determine the phenomena of human relationship and even religious faith.

The matter may best be approached by starting from the experiments on learning (74). In even very simple learning experiments, such as those on rote learning, Hull (79) has demonstrated that a phenomenon appears which is of a higher level of complexity than those which are ordinarily discussed by the psychological experimenters. It is found that an individual learning to recite nonsense syllables by rote not only learns to repeat the nonsense syllables of the given series but also becomes more skilled in learning nonsense syllables. When presented with another series of nonsense syllables, he will learn the second series more rapidly than he learned the first. Similarly, he will learn a third series more rapidly than he learned the second, and so on, up to an asymptotic limit of skill in learning nonsense syllables.

The term *"deutero-learning"* has been coined (18) to describe this higher order of learning, and this word can be regarded as a synonym for "learning to learn."

If we now consider the various sorts of learning experiments, we find that it is possible to classify the various sorts of experiments according to a formal scheme (74). There are the rote experiments, already mentioned; there are the Pavlovian experiments in which the actions of the experimental subject have no influence on the occurrence or timing of the reward or punishment; there are the instrumental reward experiments in which the subject by performing a certain act determines when the reward shall be given; there are instrumental avoidance experiments in which the subject by his own act prevents a punishing event from occurring; there are escape experiments, maze experiments, and so on. In brief, there is a series of types of time sequence and a series of different roles which can be assigned to the experimental subject; and the time sequences and the roles differ from one type of experiment to the next.

We now propose the following hypothesis for which experimental verification is not yet available: [1] if the human subject

---

[1] Since the above was written, the writer's attention has been called to Harlow's experiment on "learning sets" (72). Harlow's "learning set curves" are precisely "deutero-learning" curves.

shows the capacity for learning to learn in rote experiments, then it is likely that the phenomenon of learning to learn will occur much more widely and is, we suppose, present in all other types of learning experiments. For example, the experimental subject who has experienced a series of instrumental contexts is likely to show added skill in dealing with other instrumental contexts. In fact, there is likely to be a phenomenon of deutero-learning for each type of learning experiment: the experimental subject learning to deal with the particular type of sequential context of which he has had repeated experience.

If that is so, we may go on to ask: What sort of world will the subject with repeated experience in instrumental contexts inhabit? How will he perceive and interpret the world in which he lives? The subject will clearly expect the world to be made up of contexts appropriate for instrumental response; his threshold for the recognition of such contexts will be lowered. Similarly in regard to the Pavlovian subject we may now state that he will learn to expect a world in which he has no control over the good and evil which may befall him; he will try to know when they are coming, and he can take appropriate visceral precautions, readying his body for the food or pain. He can, so to speak, look for omens to tell him when the disaster will come, but it will not occur to him that he can do anything about the disaster, except within his own body. Similarly, the subject with repeated experience of instrumental avoidance will have a different orientation to the world from the subject with repeated experience of instrumental reward; the former looking for avoidance of punishment, the latter looking for positive gain. And so on.

Thus the discussion of the phenomena of learning moves forward from the type of question asked by psychological experimenters—"Under what circumstances will the subject learn to do such and such?"—to a higher-level question concerning the circumstances which will alter the "character structure" of the animal. The Pavlovian experimental subject becomes, as it were, a prototype for a certain species of fatalism. The subject of instrumental experiments becomes a prototype for—if you please —certain themes of American character structure; and so on.

We are, in fact, coining the beginnings of a set of formal categories for describing character structure, and these descriptions are derived not from what the subject has learned in the old simple sense of the word "learning," but from the *context* in which the simple learning occurred.

This is the level at which learning experiments become relevant to psychiatry, and the hypothesis of deutero-learning provides the bridge between simple psychology and psychiatric theory. The psychiatrist is not concerned with the question of whether the patient is able to write, to use a typewriter, to play the piano, to walk, or to do any other thing; but he is concerned with the description of the context in which the patient learned, for example, to typewrite or to control his sphincters. If the patient learned his lesson in a context of threatened punishment, that fact may throw light upon the character structure of the patient, not the mere fact of his having learned the appropriate actions.

Now, we ask, of what order is the conscious or unconscious proposition which guides the subject of instrumental experiments—the proposition which we may crudely verbalize for him as "the world is made up of contexts in which I can act instrumentally"? If we consider this statement, it is at once evident that the instrumental subject will, within certain limits, experience a world in which his propositions are apparently verified. Being an instrumental organism, he will meet the world instrumentally; he will seek out and respond to those contexts which are appropriately structured, and he will thereby reinforce his own belief that the world is an instrumental world. Correspondingly, a fatalist or Pavlovian subject, believing that he can do nothing to further his gain or avoid punishment, will act in the world in such a way that his premise about the nature of the world is demonstrated to be true. These propositions, in fact, about the world in which we live are not true or false in a simple objective sense; they are more true if we believe and act upon them, and more false if we disbelieve them. Their validity is a function of our belief.

The psychiatrist is very familiar with phenomena of this kind. The paranoid, by his action, creates about himself those relationships to human beings which will in fact reinforce his paranoid premises about the nature of human beings. If he distrusts every man and acts upon his distrust, he will find that people are remarkably untrustworthy. And the same considerations apply to a whole host of aberrational premises.

We note that the premises of which character structure is built are closely related to the contexts in which learning occurs,[2] and further that the premises of character structure are propositions of the general type which we are discussing in this chapter —namely, those whose validity depends upon the subject's belief in them.

We proceed now to discuss human relationships. In order to approach these formally while still maintaining connection with the psychological hypotheses derived from the learning experiments, it is convenient to think of the learning experiment as consisting not of an experimental subject in an inanimate environment, but as a two-person system in which the subject is face to face with another organism. We now proceed, therefore, having personified the experimental subject in the paragraphs above, to personify the experimenter. When it is bluntly stated that the experimenter is an organism, we perceive that he too has placed himself in a context of learning, more complex than that which the subject experiences. The Pavlovian subject's context is one in which he first perceives the conditioned stimulus (for example, a buzzer) and then waits a certain length of time, possibly salivating, and finally experiences the reinforcement (e.g., meat powder). If we state this whole series of events now from the point of view of the experimenter, we thereby define a complementary pattern: the experimenter first acts to give a signal (the buzzer), then remains inactive for a fixed period of time while the animal reacts in one way or another

---

[2] The precise relationship between learning to perform a given action in a certain context, which we may call *proto-learning,* and the more elaborate learning which we here call *deutero-learning* is still obscure. It is probable that all proto-learning is accompanied by at least some degree of deutero-learning, but the converse is not necessarily true. It is at least conceivable that deutero-learning may occur in entities incapable of proto-learning. In particular, Von Neumann (168) has demonstrated that certain standards and conventions of behavior must logically come into being among hypothetical competitive robots whose total rationality by hypothesis precludes all proto-learning from experience.

under his observation; and finally he administers the reinforcement, regardless of the animal's reactions. Looking at these two sides of the interaction together, we obtain paradigms for such phenomena as dominance and submission, dependency and succoring, and the like. Each of these formerly loose terms can now be sharply defined in terms of some deutero-learned premise, acquired in the learning contexts of human interaction; and these sharper definitions will discriminate a number of species of interaction which were previously confused: for example, the "dominance" of the Pavlovian experimenter is clearly different from the "dominance" of the instrumental reward experimenter.

To illustrate this it is convenient to consider the interaction between two persons, A and B, and to represent the actions of these persons by a and b respectively. With this symbolism it is possible to substitute for the loose statement "A is dependent upon B" a more precise statement, as follows: "From his past experience of interaction, A has a deutero-learned premise which leads him to expect that, in interaction with B, there will occur frequent sequences of the type:

$$a'\ b\ a''$$

where a' is a signal of weakness or need, b is B's helping or succoring response, and a'' is A's acceptance or acknowledgment of this help."

This effort at precise description may seem to the reader to be truistical, but from the study of such paradigms for dependence, succoring, dominance, submission, and the like, there emerges a curious set of paradoxes: the more sharply the paradigms are defined, the more evident it becomes that the persons concerned in the interaction actually have a curious freedom to impose their own interpretations upon the sequences of interaction. It is this freedom and its deterministic limitation by old deutero-learned premises that make it possible for the individual to perceive the sequences of interaction in his own idiosyncratic manner and so to find reinforcement for his own deutero-learned premises.

An example is necessary. The paradigm for the statement "A instrumentally dominates B" will be:

$$a'\ b\ a''$$

where a' is A's command, telling B what to do, and possibly defining the conditional reinforcement; b is B's obedient act; and a'' is A's administration of the reinforcement. Now, the paradigm for A's dominance obviously resembles the paradigm given above for A's dependence, both having the form a' b a''. The question therefore arises whether "instrumental dominance" is really different from "dependence"; or whether the participants in a given interaction have a freedom of interpretation such that a' b a'' might appear to some individuals as dominance while to others it would appear as dependence. The answer is that there are certainly many instances in which a' can be regarded either as a plea for help or as a command; similarly b can often be regarded either as a helping act or as an act of obedience; and a'', if it is a statement of acceptance, a "thank you," can be seen either as a condescending reward or as the appropriate response of the dependent. It is up to A and B each to weigh his own interpretation of the events, to determine whether A was dominant or dependent. Finally, it is important to note that A and B need not be in agreement in their perceptions at this level.

The case of Jeeves in the Wodehouse stories will provide a more concrete example. Jeeves is the elderly butler and Bertie Wooster is his scapegrace master. The question which concerns us here is whether Wooster is dependent upon Jeeves (as younger man upon older) or dominates Jeeves (as master to servant). Are Bertie's orders to the butler statements of weakness or commands? Bertie, from his side, is free to see himself as the master; but Jeeves has the freedom, from his side, to dignify his own position by seeing himself as succoring Bertie.

Thus the definition of a relationship depends not merely upon the skeleton of events which make up the interaction but also upon the way the individuals concerned see and interpret those events. This seeing or interpretation can be regarded as the application of a set of propositions about the world or the self whose validity depends upon the subject's belief in them. The individuals are partially free to interpret their world according to the premises of their respective character structure, and their freedom to do this is still further increased by the phenomena of selective awareness and by the fact that the perceiving individual plays a part in creating the appropriate sequences of action by contributing his own actions to the sequence.

In the same category with the deutero-definitions of relationship and the premises of character formation go many of the premises of any given culture. In discussing the difference between England and America (Chapter 6) it was suggested that an important fundamental difference can be derived from the fact that the child in America exhibits achievement and self-sufficiency vis-à-vis his parents, who take a spectatorship role; while in England the child takes a preponderantly spectatorship role vis-à-vis his parents, who are models showing him how to act. This American premise, that spectatorship goes along with the other characteristics of parenthood such as succoring and dominance, is not either true or false; it is a convention of the relationship, shaping character structure and owing its only validity to the unconscious or habitual acquiescence of those who participate in the relationship.

Similarly the values of American culture which have been discussed at length (Chapter 4)—puritan morality, success, change, equality, and sociability—reflect premises of this general order. The value set upon morality, success, etc., is continually reinforced by the occurrence of actions and communications in which the more abstract propositions about values are implicit. These value propositions are thus metacommunicative, and their validity depends upon the occurrence of the more concrete actions and words which result from Americans' acceptance of the values. The mechanism by which such value propositions are propagated in a culture is circular (14), (19).

Among the premises of human relationship as culturally defined, we include the premises which define the family constellation and all the premises of role and status, class and caste, which define the processes of interaction. And, in addition to all these, we have to include the conventions of international and cross-cultural conduct (13)—even the tedious and hateful conventions leading up to and ending in international warfare. Not only the premises of smooth interpersonal relationship but also the premises of hostility are carried upon the stream of more objective communication and action; and what is true of persons applies also to international relations where the gradual breakdown of a *modus vivendi* is slowly documented at a metacommunicative level. This breakdown leads ultimately to the bitter agreement upon the use of force. This agreement, however, has still the same degree of unreality or reality—the same degree of abstractness—that is characteristic of all those truths whose validity is a function of man's belief in them. If, of two nations, each comes to believe in the hostility of the other, that hostility is real to this extent and to the extent that each acts upon its belief. But it is unreal—and there is therefore always some hope for international affairs—in so far as the belief is conceivably reversible. "Tweedledum and Tweedledee *agreed* to have a battle."

This survey of propositions whose validity depends upon belief has now included within the general group of metacommunicative statements the following types: first, the propositions of codification; second, the propositions of character formation; and third, the propositions of human relationship in cultural systems. The survey will naturally continue by examining the premises of man's vast symbolic activity in the fields of play, art, and religion. It is, however, convenient to stop here to consider the bearing of current philosophical thinking upon what has been said so far.

In the preceding chapter, under the heading of contradictions in codification, it was stated that there is always a danger that an individual's lines of thought may get tangled and produce paradoxes of the general type implicit in the statement "I am lying" or in Russell's more formal problem of the "class of classes which are not members of themselves." We now face the peculiar difficulty that the discussion of metacommunication is sure to lead us into paradoxes of this very type. The construction of such paradoxes depends upon a given utterance being simultaneously a statement about itself. Taking as an example the paradox presented by the man who says, "I am lying," we are caught in paradox because he makes a statement, and he makes a statement about this statement, the second being of a different order of abstraction from the first. The paradox arises from the interplay of these two levels of abstraction.

In discussing metacommunicative propositions, we land ourselves at once in this position because metacommunicative statements are of a different level of abstraction from the simple objective statements upon the stream of which they are carried.

A considerable amount of inquiry in the last twenty years has gone into the attempt to unravel these difficulties, which came to the fore in the twenties. It was then hoped (176) that the whole of mathematics and logic might be made self-contained and unified without recourse to "self-evident" propositions, and Russell and Whitehead labored in the *Principia Mathematica* (177) to establish such a unity between mathematics and logic. It was found, however, that any such attempt involved asking, "What is really meant by the 'self-evident' axioms on which any mathematical system rests?" and that the statements which would define the axioms and give them logical foundation must always be statements of a different order of abstraction from the axioms, as the latter are contained in the theorems which are built upon them. The statements explaining the axioms are in fact metacommunicative as compared with the axioms themselves, and the latter are metacommunicative as compared with the theorems. The status of the axioms therefore becomes ambiguous, since they are used at two levels of abstraction, one relatively metacommunicative and the other relatively "objective"; and the total system of statements thus becomes comparable to the electric buzzer (p. 194) which must oscillate between the "yes" and "no" positions.

Since the days of the *Principia Mathematica* the matter has become even more difficult and more directly relevant to the questions with which we are here dealing. Gödel (63) has now demonstrated with rigorous proof that no system of statements can be self-contained in the sense of explaining its own axioms and not self-contradictory; that always—as a result of the very nature of communication and metacommunication—contradictions of the Russellian type must creep in. This statement of Gödel's—and there is apparently at present no reason to doubt his proof (176)—means in fact that psychology and the study of human communication can never hope to build a self-contained and coherent system which will not be self-contradictory.

In brief, we have to face the fact that when we deal simultaneously with both objective communication and metacommunication, contradictions will arise within the very field of our own inquiry.

In practice, this means that we must accept and must expect to find in the great creative fields of human communication—play, art, religion, epistemology, and psychiatric theory—paradoxes of the general type contained in the statement "I am lying."

We are now in a position to examine the nature of play, art, and religion. We have been warned.

In play, the element of "I am lying" is clearly recognizable. The participants in a game set up as fictions the rules of that game, they set up as a fiction (and a fluctuating fiction at that) the convention that the players are opposed to each other or are to compete with each other, and they set up fictional devices of codification to determine how gain and loss are to be symbolized. As we say, "It's only a game."

In art, the matter is more obscure but becomes clear if we consider the difference between art and propaganda (41). The propagandist is concerned with persuading his audience that what he says has more than the truth of man-made conventions. He is concerned with persuading his audience that the propagandic message is an objective statement rather than a metacommunicative message. It is true, of course, that many propagandic forms, films, plays, and the like, have an outward appearance of being honest fiction, but always in the propagandic form the accent is upon the idea that this fiction is in some sense objective truth. The story is presented as "typical," and therefore the audience is urged to act as though the play were a statement of reality. The artist, on the other hand, in contrast to the propagandist, can say honestly, "This is my creation" or "This is how I react to some part of my world"; and in this statement are contained the potentialities for paradox that occur in the statement "I am lying." The truths which the artist expresses contain frankly and honestly the combination of the metacommunicative with the objective. This is perhaps the greatest formal distinction between art and propaganda.

Similarly, Ruskin's "true" and "false" grotesque illustrates the same point. In the case of the "true" grotesque, the artist is honestly presenting some creation of the human imagination, some image either traditional or created in his own mental life, neither true nor false, but human. In the "false" grotesque, the artist tries to persuade his audience at least for a moment that his creation is a reality, is true in an objective sense, and the falsity of the false grotesque consists precisely in this—that no creation of the human imagination has this order of truth. Its only truth is that of being truly a creation—the creation of an honest mind.

In the field of religion, the problem of sorting out the objective, the propagandic, and the artistic elements, and relating these to the general category of propositions whose validity is a function of our belief in them, is exceedingly complex. Indeed, conflicting opinions about the degree of objective truth or "symbolism" contained in religious statements have been a source of strife through the centuries. The Christian religionists have notoriously tended to overstress the position that their mythologies and even parables should be regarded as objective historic truths, while the antireligionists have tended to the equally stupid opposite extreme of denying even metacommunicative or relative truth to any religious document upon which they could throw objective doubt.

Every religion has its central mythological statements. In Christianity, for example, we have the statements defining the omnipotence of God and the relationship of Father and Son to humanity. We are not concerned here with evaluating these statements at the objective or historical level. It is necessary to state, however, that whatever the degree of objective truth in the statements, they carry implicit in their poetry a large number of assertions of the type which we here discuss. We do not ask whether there *is* a Father in heaven; we only state that the words, "Our Father which art in Heaven," in addition to their objective truth or untruth, carry implicit propositions about the brotherhood of man, and we point out that these implicit propositions belong to the category which concerns us here: that, in so far as men can believe and act upon their imputed brotherhood, this premise will determine their mutual relations; and that in so far as they disbelieve and act upon their disbelief, the implicit contrary proposition becomes true.

The preceding paragraphs raise questions which cannot be answered as yet—especially the question regarding the limits of deutero-truth. We state that the validity of a deutero-proposition *is a function of* belief, and it is clear enough that in many instances there is a range of values for the variables "validity" and "belief" in which an increase of belief will be accompanied by increase of validity. But this is very far from saying that the relationship between these variables is linear or that total belief will be accompanied by total validity. Indeed, it is probable that total validity can only be reached in special instances—if ever. More usually (e.g., in the case of the brotherhood of man) we may expect the validity of the proposition to reach a maximum beyond which future increases of belief will result in frustrating experiences for the believers, some of whom will then doubt the validity of the proposition. Further complications will follow if there is a division of opinion in a population, and that particular species of conflict is likely to occur which Collingwood has described as "eristic"—i.e., conflict about some variable which, if let alone, would settle itself at a value intermediate between the values for which the two sides strive.

The occurrence of such deutero-propositions throughout the fabric of every religious system can only be mentioned. It must, however, be stated that truths of the sort which we discuss are implicit in all religious communication, whether it is mythology or ritual, and that these propositions include not only the ethical implications of religion for human action but also the theories which any particular religion uses to define the relationship between man and the universe. Religion (25) is the great storehouse of those deutero-learned propositions which are summarized in such words as "fatalism," "instrumentalism," "passivity," "acquiescence," "free will," "determinism," "responsibility," "guilt," acceptance of the universe or revolt against it, and so on.

In fact, religion, like science and philosophy and art, is one of the mass agencies which determine our epistemology—our theories of the nature of the reality in which we live and our theories of the nature of our knowledge of this reality.

This brings us to the conclusion of this chapter. In the next chapter the epistemology implicit in a collection of psychiatric statements will be examined. In contrast, the previous chapter and the present discussion of deutero-propositions form, together, a statement of the epistemology of the authors. This is the definition of our point of view, from which we shall study the psychiatrist's statements. And this statement of the authors' position must be concluded upon a strange negative note. As was said above, it seems that all attempts to build a coherent body of statements at several levels of abstraction must always end in paradox and contradiction. It is evident that statements about the theory of knowing are exceedingly abstract and are members of the class of propositions whose validity depends in part upon belief. This would indicate that the actual processes of knowledge (like the processes of learning discussed above) are surely modified by the knower's theory of the nature of knowledge. If this is so, then there must be a limit beyond which epistemology cannot go—a limit at which our attempt to resolve the contradictions of experience and communication will break down.

At the time of writing, the last word which must be added to the description of the authors' epistemological position is an acknowledgment that we expect our own position, like all others, to be, in the end, either incomplete or self-contradictory.

9 · PSYCHIATRIC THINKING: An Epistemological Approach

By Gregory Bateson

TRADITIONALLY, "epistemology" means the theory of knowledge —the study of the nature of knowing—and the branch of philosophy which has grown up around the word is intertwined with ontology, the study of the nature of being. Indeed, Descartes' famous *"cogito ergo sum"*—"I think, therefore I am"— defines a meeting point of these two types of philosophical inquiry.

In the preceding chapter, an attempt was made to state the authors' epistemological position; and in the course of the statement, the very meaning of the word "epistemology" was changed from the conventional. It was argued that the study of knowing or, as we call it, the study of "information," is inseparable from the study of communication, codification, purpose, and values. We have thus modified the study of epistemology towards the inclusion of a specific range of external phenomena, and at the same time have shifted the subject in our handling of it somewhat away from philosophical abstractions and toward scientific generalization.

In the present chapter we use the word "epistemology" in this latter sense and attempt to describe the epistemology which guides contemporary American psychiatric thinking and utterance.

Now, to a large number of psychiatrists of the present day, "epistemology" has not this more scientific and less philosophical meaning. If they use the word at all, they do so in the narrower and more conventional sense of "theory of knowledge." Our task, therefore, is to describe as best we may the premises upon which psychiatrists think and speak, and to do so within the framework of our own epistemological premises.

At an earlier stage of this book, we argued that only where there is difference between two persons in contact is it possible for those persons to achieve a new understanding, a new awareness of the previously unconscious premises which underlie their own habits of communication. The same, we believe, is true of epistemologies: that if A wishes to study the epistemology of B, he can do so only if his own epistemology differs from that of B to such an extent that he is driven to some awareness of his own and of B's premises. And even with the help of difference and contrast, the task will still be difficult: The present chapter can only be a crude preliminary attempt at a well-nigh impossible task.

Our subject matter, also, is fraught with emotional charges and controversial implications. These must be faced frankly if communication is to occur. An epistemology, after all, is like a scientific theory or hypothesis. Like any other theory it can be a focus of controversy in which the winning side is likely to associate certain feelings of superiority with the winning. But an epistemology is also like a scientific theory in that it is never right. It is at best, and however well it works, only a working hypothesis, subject to future correction and change. The scientist may do the best he can, but he can never, in the nature of the case, achieve a theory which is not subject to disproof. Always the undiscovered facts and the ongoing changes in the climate of scientific thought will have the last word—the scientist never.

There is another difficulty which besets the present study: the authors at the moment of writing have arrived at a particular epistemological position, but, from this single position, which we have tried to make coherent, we have to view a vast variety of positions—a mixture of coherence and incoherence. Among psychiatrists today, some habitually think in disciplined Aristotelian terms, i.e., in an epistemology laid down in classical Athens; others try to think with rigor in an epistemology more comparable to that of Wiener or of Korzybski; others again—and these are the majority—do not worry about questions of epistemology, and in their utterances there is implicit a complex mixture of epistemological premises derived from all stages of Occidental thought in the last two thousand years.

We do not, any of us, achieve rigor. In writing, sometimes, we can take time to check the looseness of thought; but in speaking, hardly ever. It is exceedingly difficult in conversation to say what one means, and rarely does one speak consistently in terms of a single epistemology. This comparative looseness of the spoken word is mentioned because the data used in this inquiry are for the most part the spoken words of psychiatrists in informal conversation. What they said was often not their considered utterance; they spoke as they would not if they were writing in a formal context. I know that I personally, when speaking in conversation and even in lecturing, depart continually from the epistemology outlined in the previous chapter; and indeed that chapter itself was hard to write without continual lapses into other ways of thinking and may still contain such lapses. I know that I would not like to be held scientifically responsible for many loose spoken sentences that I have uttered in conversation with scientific colleagues. But I also know that if another person had the task of studying my ways of thought, he would do well to study my loosely spoken words rather than my writing.

For these reasons, the reader is asked to remember this: that most of the utterances of psychiatrists quoted in this chapter are not their serious and considered scientific pronouncements but are rather straws in the wind which indicate how the speakers think—often gropingly—between one scientific pronouncement and another. Moreover, the samples are specimens of speech and, while the forms and syntax and metaphors of speech are undoubtedly coercive upon the ways of thought of the speaker (96), (184), there is not a one-to-one relation between thought and speech. It may often happen that a speaker would, if he could, speak in terms of a more flexible or more sophisticated epistemology, but finds himself restricted by the language forms which are current in his culture and epoch. In this chapter, however, we shall ignore this possible discrepancy between thought and speech, perhaps with some injustice to the speakers. Our aim, after all, is to describe just those very limitations of psychiatric thought which are characteristic of the subculture of psychiatrists in this epoch. In the following chapter an attempt will be made to discuss trends in psychiatric thinking, and in this connection the discrepancy between the budding ideas of tomorrow and the language of today will be discussed. For the rest we hope that the speakers will not feel hurt because they are quoted as human beings, creatures of an epoch and liable to err, rather than as precise utterers of rigorous theory.

The plan of description will be as follows:

We shall first discuss, one by one, a series of notions which recur commonly in the utterances of psychiatrists—their assumptions about pathology, reality, substance, energy, quantification, and the reflexive nature of their science. Treating these items separately will of course be a falsification, because a man's epistemology is not made up of separable items: it is a unitary and complex system which underlies his thought and speech. The falsification of dealing with the items separately is, however, necessary in order to reduce the subject of our discussion into manageable pieces. Moreover, this treatment of separate items will make it difficult for the reader to appreciate the progressive change and flux of psychiatric thinking: the time dimension will be lacking. In order to add this missing dimension, the following chapter will be an essay upon the trends in current psychiatric epistemology.

We now proceed to discuss five epistemological notions, one by one, as though they were separate items.

PATHOLOGY

Psychiatry has grown up as a study of pathology, and the view which contemporary psychiatrists take of this science of pathology may be illustrated by a statement quoted from one of them. He divides the history of psychiatry into three periods, the descriptive, the epithetic, and the thematic, and he describes these periods as follows: "In the period of *descriptive* psychiatry the psychiatrist used to be referred to as an 'alienist,' that is, as a person who is interested in strange behavior. . . . The *epi-thetic* stage of psychiatry . . . when the psychiatrist was interested in kinds of persons—'introvert,' 'seclusive,' 'schizoid,' and so on. These are adjectival categories and the emotional attitude [of the psychiatrist] made these adjectives into epithets. *Thematic* psychiatry is a later stage. It is the study of the themes or issues which are important to the patient, both within the period of morbidity and in the premorbid period. These three levels [descriptive, epithetic, and thematic] are all proper and necessary today. There may be some disdain for the descriptive and the epithetic, but all three levels are still necessary."

Perhaps as a residue from the descriptive and epithetic periods, the terminology of psychiatry is on the whole rich in words describing the undesirable and abnormal and is impoverished in regard to words which would describe the desirable and the healthy. The tendency toward specialization in the abnormal is modified in various ways; but for the moment we discuss only the fact of emphasis upon the abnormal and note that even within the domain of psychiatry, the practitioners and therapists often regret that their science is a science of the abnormal. They urge one another to study the normal.

The psychiatric emphasis upon the abnormal is dramatically evident to anybody who works in a neighboring science such as psychology or anthropology. We in the neighboring sciences look to the psychiatrists for terms and ideas which can be applied in our fields. In anthropology, for example, there is a tendency to borrow the terms of psychiatric diagnosis for the description of human beings in other cultures. The Germans are described as "paranoid"; the Japanese culture is diagnosed by its anal emphasis; Balinese culture is somehow related to "schizophrenia"; and so on.

Be all that as it may, for the moment we disregard the impacts on other sciences and are concerned with reasons why the language of psychiatry should stress the abnormal and with the implications of this. First, there is the fact of therapy: the patient is different—or feels himself to be different—from the remainder of the population; he comes to have this difference modified or to be made able to accept it. But this alone would not be sufficient to determine the characteristic which we are discussing. If, for example, it were effective to tell the patient about normality, the language of psychiatry would surely have developed a rich terminology for this type of educational therapy. That it has not done so is due to a variety of circumstances— not merely the impossibility of "telling the patient," but also a belief on the part of the psychiatrists that the healthy state toward which patient A might progress is certain to be unique for him, and that of patients B, C, and D, each will have his own unique possibilities for growth and development. Language can only deal with recurring phenomena; never can it specify the unique, and especially the uniquely personal developments and complex growth which are still in the future. It would appear that the phenomena of pathology are actually simpler, more general, and more recurrent than those of normality and health.

Moreover, according to the general theory outlined in the preceding chapter, organisms are to be regarded as self-corrective entities. If this hypothesis is correct, then the information which an organism mainly needs is data about its errors and about those conditions in the external world which threaten survival or cause discomfort. Whatever area of human life we look at, we find that the vocabulary is rich for describing appetites, dissatisfactions, discomforts, and the like, and rich for the description of the instrumentalities to correct these conditions. But in all areas of life, the vocabulary is on the whole poor in words which define states of relaxation, satisfaction, and low tension; and poor in words to describe satisfactory conditions in the external world. We can say that we are hot or cold in a vast variety of idiom and metaphor, but to say that the temperature of the body is just right we have but few words. I remember vividly the pleasant feeling of cultural shock which accompanied the discovery that the Balinese language contains a word, *tis*, for that state of body temperature which is just right, the feeling neither hot nor cold, the feeling of smooth relaxation which follows sexual intercourse (22).

A similar specialization in the analysis of the undesirable can be recognized also, to cite another example, in the field of aesthetics. The art critic is much more able to say what is wrong with a picture or musical composition than he is able to express appreciation. Indeed, he often relapses into inarticulateness and incoherence when he tries to say what he admires or enjoys.

It is true that human beings, besides being self-corrective and avoiding the unpleasant and painful, are also pleasure-seeking, and the position of pleasure in psychiatric thinking will be discussed later. For the present we observe that psychiatry is preponderantly concerned with the perception and description of the abnormal and undesirable and that the technical vocabulary is almost entirely focused upon the pathological aspects. Many psychiatrists, in fact, complete their training without becoming familiar with some of the most fundamental ideas in the related but non-normative science of psychology.

Moreover, the thinking of psychiatrists on the subject of pathology is rendered more complex and even paradoxical by two trends: (a) the tendency to doubt the reality of "clinical entities," and (b) the insistence that the patient's symptoms are indications of life and health because they are his spontaneous efforts to cure himself. The symptoms are efforts at self-corrective change, even though such self-correction may be inept.

Three quotations from psychiatrists will serve to illustrate this shift of emphasis away from the clinical entity and towards the focus upon mechanisms of "defense":

A Freudian analyst says: "Freud's nosology is poor, and [for example] hysteria does not appear as an entity. Rather, Freud is concerned with assigning etiology. The overt [symptoms] which you can put down are not the criteria, but it is 'hysteria' if the symptoms originate in repressed early childhood sexual impulse and if the defenses involve somatic function in symbolic form."

And on another occasion, the same speaker states: "There is no such thing as *a* mental illness. There are only mechanisms of a neurotic or psychotic nature. Normality includes all possible neurotic and psychotic mechanisms. If none are predominant and all are under the individual's control, he is 'normal.'"

Another Freudian states: "Neurosis is the expression of a tendency to repeat the experience and master the stimulus by repetition," and "If the child is capable of accepting the conditions and mastering traumatic events by repetition, then he is normal."

A Jungian similarly shifts emphasis away from the clinical entity, but where the Freudians stress etiology, he stresses prognosis. Describing the initial interview, he says: "I look at the psychiatric [not the typological] aspects of the case—but see them not as a diagnosis—rather as prognosis. It is not a case history but a talk; and on the basis of his demands I see whether I think I can help."

The matter becomes even more complex when a sociological or cultural dimension is added to the concepts of pathology. For example, in discussing the problem of delinquency, a Freudian analyst states: "I would not start with the person who is 'at fault' but with the persons who define what is a fault. We should ask, 'Why does *who* call it a crime?' "

This discussion of psychiatry as a science of pathology points up sharply the outcome of attempting to compare the epistemology of psychiatry with that of the writers. What has been argued above amounts to this, that a characteristic of psychiatry which the psychiatrists themselves recognize and sometimes lament appears to be one which, arguing from the writer's epistemological position, is to be expected. If the very nature of the communications process is such that it must in the main be concerned with self-correction; if it lies in the very nature of this process that only recurrent phenomena can be discussed; and if the phenomena of abnormality are simpler and more recurrent than the unique complex and varied phenomena of health—then the position which has developed in psychiatry is one which is to be expected.

The only unexpected item is the comparative lack of terminology and articulate statement to deal with the instrumentalities of therapy. The psychiatrists are short of words to describe the implementation of their task. Very little has been done to specify the tricks and recipes of therapy. Indeed, it is a common complaint of young psychiatric residents and others who apprentice themselves to the profession that their teachers cannot tell them what to do.

In sum, it is a science rather inarticulate about its operations and with its theoretical focus concentrated upon the diagnosis of abnormality and the analysis of normal dynamics in abnormal circumstances. The dynamics of normal circumstance and the methods of implementing the therapeutic process are comparatively little studied. The exceptions to this general statement must, however, be mentioned.

As regards the specification of methods in therapy, it is worth remarking that the chief attempts in this direction occur in those schools and branches of psychotherapy where the process of therapy is most seen as akin to an engineering process. The general poverty of terminology and recipes to define procedures in psychotherapy probably results partly, as mentioned above, from the lack of specificity in the goals towards which therapy works. But the notion that the goals of life and health cannot be specified is itself an epistemological premise. In particular it is a notion which is surely historically connected with the European origin of the principal schools of psychiatric thought. America is notoriously the land of "know-how." American culture stresses—almost as though it were an item of religious dogma—the notion that goals can be specified and that the means of attaining those goals can then be planned with articulate clearness. In general, Europeans hardly believe this; their goals are related to an ongoing normalcy rather than to specific achievement.

Culture contact between America and Europe leads to strange blendings and contrasts. A European-born psychiatrist says: "There is a sort of *opportunism of health*. After successful therapy, the patient continues to use this opportunism as a test of what he wants to do, a test of values." But in reply to the words "opportunism of health," an American-born Freudian makes a wry face and says that the phrase reminds him of the title of a recent book on William Blake, *The Politics of Vision*.

It may clarify this problem of culture contact to add, for the benefit of American readers, an Englishman's note on the difference between the words "British" and "English." In the United Kingdom, there are many cultural systems: English, Irish, Scots, Welsh, and many smaller regional systems. These are politically lumped together under the general term "British." Because of this political aspect and because the local intricacies of pattern are blurred when all are classified together, the term "British" has come to denote a frame of mind oriented to more specific goals, while the regional terms denote views of the world which do not have this jingoistic and expansionist flavor. It would appear that culture contact—whether it be in Britain or in the American "melting pot"—is a phenomenon which influences human beings toward a habit of specific goal orientation and away from the richer habitual participation in the maintenance of intricate patterns. Thus the term "British" denotes that outward mask of the British subject in which he appears as a product of culture contact, but under the skin of every "Britisher"—even the most brash—there is an Englishman or an Irishman or a Scot or a Yorkshireman, whose more intimate values are the intricacy of his special regional culture. In this sense, the whole problem of goal orientation in American psychiatry is related to the conflict between culture-contacted and goal-oriented man on the one side and culturally intact, pattern-oriented man on the other.

Returning to the psychiatric scene, we note that it is in those variants of psychiatric procedure which have been developed in America that the greatest efforts have been made to specify the methods of operation. Examples are to be seen in the "non-directional" therapy of Rogers, in narcosynthesis, in the hypnotic techniques of Milton Erickson, Brenman and Gill, and so on. And perhaps the newest development, Dianetics (78), should be mentioned in this connection as a type of therapy devised by an electronic engineer who makes a definite attempt to introduce engineering "know-how" into psychiatric procedure.

In all these developments, we observe American culture patterns impacting upon systems of preponderantly European origin. In fact, we can trace here a deep conflict of values and epistemology—a conflict between that view of the world in which the ultimate values are presumed to be complex and unspecifiable and a view of the world which assumes that the ultimate human values can at any given moment be specified in terms of definite goals. The outcome of this conflict lies still in the future, but it is possible to relate the conflict to current trends in the epistemology of psychiatry.

REALITY

We may introduce the discussion of reality by quoting the words of a Freudian lecturer, replying to a question from the floor. He said: "Yes. In fact, I wanted to come to that. In fact, . . . I have to modify again everything I said." The concept "reality" is slippery because, always, truth is relative to context, and context is determined by the questions which we ask of events.

Inevitably the concept of reality has a double face, so that every reference to "reality" is ambiguous. We can never be quite clear whether we are referring to the world as it *is* or to the world as we *see* it. This ambiguity affects theoretical thinking in psychology and psychiatry and affects also the ethical and moral precepts implicit or explicit in therapy. Indeed, the only way of maintaining some clarity in philosophical and psychological statement is to be aware of the inevitable ambiguity. And yet it is hard or impossible to imagine a scientific psychiatry which would not, in the end, invoke some concept of reality.

Broadly, there are five common uses of the word "reality" in psychiatric utterance:

A. The word "reality" is used to denote the external world as perceived via the senses. Using the word in this sense, the speaker assumes the simplicity and credibility of sense data, and blurs the fact that these data are to be interpreted in ways which conform to his own and other people's interpretations. In this sense the word "reality" is opposed to such words as "fantasy" on the one hand and "projection" on the other—where "fantasy" refers to products of the inner stream of psychic life, and "projection" refers to the results of idiosyncratic perception, especially when the idiosyncrasy is unrecognized.

The following quotations from psychiatrists illustrate this use of the concept:

A Jungian: "Reality implies minimal projection."

A Freudian: "The only goal of analysis is clarification of what the patient perceives—a change in his perception."

Another psychiatrist: "The perception of things outside may be wrong. Or the actions may be wrong. Or the feelings may be wrongly perceived."

B. The word "reality" is used by psychiatrists in a way which seems, superficially, to be the exact contrary of the way described above. As a result, perhaps, of the spread of relativistic habits of thought (such theories as, for example, that of "cultural relativity," according to which the interpretation of the same events is likely to be different from one culture to another), psychiatrists are beginning to speak of every individual as having his own unique "reality," his "private world."

A Jungian: "When I look at a light, I assume that the 'lightness' is within myself—that I project it upon the lamp."

Another Jungian (speaking about a patient with great creative ability to whom an important artistic assignment was offered): "She said, 'But this has nothing to do with me. I don't know why these things happen to me.' It's just as though she had no connection with it at all. So, of course, she doesn't go on with any of it. She does all these things—but there is no reality anywhere. So that, to become adapted, from page one, is her problem—to discover what happens in human relationships. Her mythologies are all Platonic images of what, for example, friendship or love might be."

C. The word "reality" is used in a third way which, in some degree, resolves the contrast between the first and second. If a man has his own idiosyncratic view of himself and the world in which he lives, this fact can be regarded as a part of "reality." He can become aware that he has this idiosyncratic view. With this awareness he is *ipso facto* in possession of more information and is therefore in a more favorable position to act adaptively or purposively in the world. He can, in some sense, transcend his unique reality and operate in terms of a reality one degree more abstract. He can "correct for" his private views, or he can "allow for" the circumstance that others do not see the world as he does.

By accepting the peculiarities of his own mental processes, a man achieves a freedom to correct for these peculiarities. This we may refer to as the *adjustive* theory of therapy—the theory that a man's peculiar habits of special interpretation are never or not immediately dropped in the therapeutic process but that they persist with the addition of new psychic habits. He may develop the additional habit of taking every conclusion which he reaches and performing upon it a further computational process which will correct for his known habitual errors.

To cite an example from personal experience: I sometimes have the experience of disorientation upon coming up into the street from the subway. I have the intuitive sense that I am facing north when, in fact, I am facing south. Moving in accordance with this intuition, I soon observe that the street numbers indicate that I am moving in the opposite direction to that which I intend. The intuitive sense remains unchanged, but I now have knowledge of what I am doing and know that to get to my destination I have only to do the opposite of what my intuition tells me. To obey this intellectual premise which runs counter to intuition evokes some anxiety, but after doing so for a few minutes I find that the intuition has corrected itself. By analogy, it would appear that the adjustive theory, if patient and therapist act in accordance with it, may lead to deeper changes in the latter's perception—perhaps by some tendency of the mind to economize and shorten its own paths of computation (187) by a canceling out of both the initial habit of distortion and the later habit of correction.

To illustrate this concept of reality we quote:

A Jungian: "To know what type you belong to should give a sort of freedom—a power to be no longer completely bound by that type."

A Freudian: "Diagnosis . . . a seeing through symptoms to the real nature of the disease. . . . It is the province and obligation of the physician to diagnose. It is basically for diagnosis that the patient comes to the doctor. . . . Once diagnosis is made, the doctor is relatively inactive. . . . Cure depends upon the patient's willingness to meet the demands of reality as stated in the diagnosis."

D. The word "reality" is used in a fourth sense which is only indirectly and by inadvertence associated with the first three. This sense appears commonly in the phrase "the reality principle," which "principle" is commonly contrasted with "the pleasure principle," giving to the word "reality" a special valuational flavor of discipline or unpleasure. Here the term "reality" slips from referring to that which exists or that which is perceived, and comes to refer to a world of values. And the link between the first three uses and this fourth use is perhaps related to the point which was stressed in the preceding chapter, that in the writer's epistemology perception and evaluation are closely overlapping concepts.

Further, the "reality principle" and the "pleasure principle" seem to be related to time perspective. A Freudian puts the matter very bluntly in these words: "The psyche is born when the child becomes capable of postponing or inhibiting discharge— when the baby learns to wait—or begins to wait—when he recognizes that preparations are being made to relieve his tensions."

And again the same assumption that "reality" is related to the longer time perspectives rather than to immediate pleasures is implicit in the following statement by a Freudian who was discussing the qualifications necessary in an analyst. He said that the candidate "should be able to work on a job as a problem, and be able to forgo the gratifications readily available between any two people."

Similarly a given action is likely to be labeled by psychiatrists as motivated in terms of (pre-logical) "pleasure" or in terms of "reality" according to whether it leads to immediate or to deferred gratification; but this relation to time is unclear and is not conventionally stated in this blunt form. After all, motivation may spring from the desire to survive as well as from pleasure-pain; and survival motivations are included under the "reality principle," being perhaps the very core of this principle. The overlap between "survival" and "deferred gratification" is easy to understand, since the man who plans deferred gratification must of necessity plan to survive longer in order to enjoy that to which he looks forward.

Finally, the overlap between these "reality" motivations and the uses of the term "reality" to refer to a perceived universe follows from the circumstance that he who would survive long and achieve deferred goals in a human community is under some necessity of either perceiving the human universe as his fellows perceive it, or of knowing how his own perceptions differ from theirs.

E. The word "reality" is used in contrast to such words as "magic," and here there is an area of considerable confusion due in part to defining "reality" in pragmatic instead of objective or epistemological terms. A Jungian states: "Reality is what works—but that won't do. It's not good enough. Though, in the long run, nothing but reality does work."

The trouble arises from the undoubted fact that magic has certain effects, especially upon him who practices it, and therefore magic cannot be discarded or overlooked as an element in an egocentronic universe. And yet, the value which Freud placed upon the rational ego raised this entity to a pinnacle from which all the "magic" of human life sometimes appeared unreal. The following excerpts from a discussion of these matters among several Freudians will serve as illustration:

1st Freudian: "Quacks consciously encourage magical thinking. We have to distinguish between rational treatment, which is the task of a psychoanalyst, and mere magical healing."

2nd Freudian: "It is true that the gullibility of the patient is used by the quack. But *faith* also is normal and necessary—a feeling of being loved and an expectation that this love will satisfy a need. . . . The psychoanalyst works, not rationally, but magically. Faith is an unavoidable component of human nature and should be utilized."

3rd Freudian: "Can we discountenance magic? . . . How much do we know concerning the effect of the psyche upon the organism?"

2nd Freudian: "Love is a pre-realistic and pre-logical function—it is not based on egocentronic thinking."

1st Freudian: "It is a demand of *reality* that love exist in the world."

The writer's opinion on these matters has been outlined in the preceding chapter. I believe that some of the difficulties disappear when we say that faith is an acceptance of deutero-propositions whose validity is *really* increased by our acceptance of them.

SUBSTANCES IN PSYCHIATRY

One of the most interesting tangles in Occidental thought is that which has grown up around the words "form" and "substance," and this tangle recurs as an element in psychiatric theory. Traditionally, in the line of thought which runs down from Aristotle through St. Thomas Aquinas to the present day, "substance" is that in which qualities are inherent, that which "sub-stands" or supports the qualities. Thus, when we say that "the lemon is yellow," it is implied that yellowness exists. The yellowness is therefore somehow separable from the "substance" of the lemon with which it is yet in some way linked. "Substance," according to this line of argument, is regarded as not itself having qualities (not even the quality of substantiality). Thus to one who believes in transubstantiation in the Sacrament of the Mass, it is not disturbing that the contents of the chalice, after transubstantiation into the Blood, do not show the physical and chemical attributes of blood. According to orthodox belief, only the substance is changed, not the qualities.

In the present context, these ancient arguments will not be resolved, but it is necessary to indicate the position which the authors take and from that position to discuss how the traditional controversies are implicit in modern psychiatric thinking.

Influenced by the thinking of Whitehead (178), we would regard the paradoxes of "form" and "substance" as probably derivative from the subject-predicate relation. Translating this view of Whitehead's into the terminology of communications theory, we would say that the subject-predicate relation is a premise or rule of Indo-European linguistic codification.[1] We

[1] The separation between subject and attribute, and in general the notion of qualities as separable from substantives, is not a necessary characteristic of language and indeed does not occur in all existing languages. For example, Dorothy Lee (96) discusses the fact that the Trobriand language has not this characteristic. The Trobriand language has no words that Dr. Lee is willing to regard as adjectives, but instead, it has a very large supply of highly differentiated substantival forms. It is thus possible for the Trobriand speaker to do without the adjectives "ripe" and "unripe" because he uses one substantive for "unripe yam" and another for "ripe yam." In fact, not only does he "do without" the adjectival form, he even does not think of qualities as conceivably separable from the substantives because he has not the idea of what an adjective is. In Latin, also, it is impossible

would argue that the statement of such a premise or rule of codification is not information about the relation between the "yellowness" and the "substance" of the lemon, but rather that the statement of the rule is information about the relation between the speaker and the lemon.

From this point of view we would regard the whole cycle of form-and-substance paradoxes as resulting from a confusion of levels of abstraction. A statement of a rule of codification is at one level of abstraction, and a statement about the lemon is at another. To draw from the linguistic form conclusions about the relation between the lemon and its yellowness is to mix these levels of abstraction. If in language we separate attributes from substance, this is not an indication that any such separation "really" occurs.

Turning now to the psychiatrists, we find that the problems of "substance" were encountered by Freud and that, as an Occidental thinker of the nineteenth century, he naturally followed the traditional line of Aristotelian-Thomist thinking. In America today this line of thinking is less fashionable and is perhaps becoming incomprehensible to the younger generation. The writer was present on one occasion when a number of young American psychiatrists attended a lecture by a Central European scholar on the history of the Freudian ideas. The lecturer dealt with the history of the concept "libido." He pointed out that this concept was derived by Freud from the study of individual life histories, approximately as follows: in an adult individual, there occur various activities, political, professional, social, sexual, and so on. These activities can be traced back and it can be shown that the activities of today have replaced, or have been evolved from, other earlier activities. In this way it is possible to trace a sort of genealogical tree of activities going backwards into infancy. The lecturer stated that the term "sexuality" as used by Freud refers collectively to all those activities

---

to use a verb without including in the very word which denotes action some reference to the agent. "*Cogito*" is translated into English as "I think," but clearly a violence is here done: the stated relation between the person and the act of thought is changed. "*Cogito ergo sum,*" a central dictum of epistemology, is only doubtfully translatable into the English language.

of the individual which can be derived, in this sense, from thumbsucking in the infant.

Freud saw that there was change; that the activities replace one another through life; and he felt that it was necessary to postulate something as continuing in order that he might speak about changes. We say that litmus paper changes from blue to red, and in order to speak of the change we find it necessary to refer to some substantive—the paper or the dye—which continues throughout the change or, as we say, "undergoes" the change, something, itself neither red nor blue, but in which the change from red to blue occurs. Similarly Freud postulated "libido" in order to have a substantive which would undergo the changes which he observed in psychosexual life.

In this thinking, Freud was evidently following passively the Aristotelian-Thomist habit. What is interesting is that the audience of young American psychiatrists was puzzled. It is true that our language still carries on the habit of separating subject from predicate, substance from attribute, but apparently in spite of this continuing linguistic habit, the sophisticated thought that lay behind Freud's early postulation of the libido is partly outdated.

Such a loss of sophistication is certainly to be regretted. The theory of substance, after all, helped to keep the rules of codification straight by stressing the fact that every attribution of a form or quality was *only* an attribution. Without some equivalent rule, speakers continually fall into semantic errors, and not infrequently end up with a complete distrust of language.

Some examples will make this clear:

A Freudian: "The generalized metaphor always kills. Congress, for example, is a tremendously interesting institution, but, when reduced to the sort of terms that an anthropologist might use, for example, to a diagrammatic repeat of the American family structure, it loses all interest."

A Jungian: "I don't go about it (case history taking) systematically. Much more comes gradually. It is like a character in a novel which comes to life gradually. Otherwise he is *only* a type."

A Freudian: "The accuracy of the report kills imagination.

I would rather you had an imaginative report of what I said."

A Freudian: "The more experience I have in psychiatry, the more convinced I become that it is impossible to verbalize what I do."

Indeed, psychiatrists—and especially the more gifted and imaginative members of the profession—devote not a little of their time to moaning that "the letter killeth"; and the development of their science is not a little delayed by their unwillingness to take notes upon what happens in therapy. All of this protest against the "letter" is, it seems to the writer, related to fallacies of codification, and especially to that fallacy which equates the codified message with that to which it refers. If, in Korzybski's phrase, we confuse the "map" with the "territory," then indeed the cartographer has killed the territory for us: he has destroyed our imagination and bound us into his little symbols on paper so that we shall never again see the landscape. If we believe that the complex institution "Congress" *is* the diagram drawn by an anthropologist, then we shall naturally distrust all such diagrams. If, on the other hand, the rules of codification are kept clear and the diagram is seen for what it is, namely an attempt at external codification of an idea in an anthropologist's head, then no harm is done.

It seems that there are several possible positions which we may take: the classical position is that taken by Freud, who separated "substance" from its attributes and let it stand as a device of codification. Second, there is the position taken by those who confuse map with territory and land in all the fallacies of false concreteness—treating the libido as a causal entity instead of a linguistic device. Third, there is the position of those who protest against all map making and all attempts at precision because they must repudiate the fallacies of the second position. Lastly, there is a possible position in which again the devices of codification, such as the separation of substance and attribute, would be accepted as simply devices of codification.

ENERGY AND QUANTIFICATION

This subject may be introduced by a series of quotations, all of them from Freudian analysts.

" 'Energy'—this was a pseudo-term. He (Freud) thought it would be some sort of energy but it might also be some spatial arrangement in the body."

"Freud also has an economic point of view, defining the tendency to keep levels of excitement at a minimum. . . . Sudden rises must be painful."

"Repressed material . . . is like a foreign body in the psyche and presses for discharge . . . it may reach expression in derivative forms."

"From a neurophysiological point of view, a neurosis is an expression of the efforts of a repressed stimulus to achieve discharge. It is an energy break in the wall between consciousness and the unconscious."

Around the concept of "energy" Freud and his followers have constructed theories which they themselves have compared to the theories of nineteenth-century economics. The foundations of psychoanalysis were laid in the same scientific period with the theories of classical economics, and both alike reflect the physics of the 1850's. In that period, the law of the conservation of energy (the First Law of Thermodynamics) formulated by Mayer in 1840 and by Joule in 1845 dominated the trends of orthodox thought. It is not relevant to the present discussion to ask how much the physical theories of the day had to do with the shaping either of economics or of psychoanalytic theory. We note only that in all three fields a similar trend occurs, and even that related trends of thought dominated biology in the same period and that these led to the theory of natural selection and to such notions as that the male is preponderantly catabolic while the female is anabolic.

It is also important that the whole train of thought connected with the Second Law of Thermodynamics (Carnot, 1824; Clausius, 1850; Clerk Maxwell, 1831–1879; Willard Gibbs, 1876; Wiener, *Cybernetics*, 1948) is ignored by psychiatrists to the extent that while the word "energy" is daily on their lips, the word "entropy" is almost unknown to them. Perhaps if they had followed Freud's alternative notion of a "spatial arrangement," mentioned in the first quotation above, the present state of theory would be more coherent.

It is not, however, the task of the present survey to criticize the Freudian theories. This has been done already by Kubie, himself a Freudian practitioner (94). Rather, we attempt two tasks: first, we seek to make clear how the Freudian system of energy phrasings is related to the general theory of communication here proposed; and second, we attempt to understand the deutero-implications of the Freudian theories. Granting that the Freudians and many other psychiatrists still think in these ways in the twentieth century (61), how will this affect their therapeutic operations and social values?

The Freudian energy theories have four main types of content:

A. Psychic energy is related to but not synonymous with such concepts as motivation, drive, purpose, wish, love, hate, and the like. The exact nature of the relationship between psychic energy and motivation is unclear, but it seems that psychic energy is a "substance" (in the strict sense) whose phenomenal aspect is motivation. Psychic energy has its sources in the deep instinctual systems of the personality.

B. Psychic energy is indestructible.

C. Psychic energy is protean in its transformations, so that a wish or hatred not acted upon in one way will predictably find phenomenal expression in some other way. Sublimation is an example of such transformation of energy.

D. Psychic energy is limited in quantity, and the total quantity available in a given organism is of the same order as the quantity needed by the organism for motivating the multiple activities of life. If, for example, much energy is wasted in psychic conflict, the organism will thereby be impoverished.

Historically, Freud and the philosophers of the nineteenth century knew of no physical model from which they could derive a precise formulation of the nature of purpose. They failed to perceive the formal analogy between the self-corrective characteristics of the internal environment (then being documented by Claude Bernard) and the self-corrective phenomena of adaptive behavior and purpose. Indeed, it was the unsolved problems of teleology that determined the great historic gulf between the natural sciences and the sciences of man. It seems that Freud's energy theories were an attempt to bridge this gulf by borrowing from physics the concept of energy and partially equating this concept with motivation. (The theory of natural selection was another attempt of the same kind.)

Today there exist many physical and biological models which exhibit self-corrective characteristics—notably the servomechanisms (134), the ecological systems (80), and the homeostatic systems (37)—and we know a great deal about the working and the limitations of models of this kind (153). The entire problem of teleology is therefore changed, and today it is evident that a bridge between the natural and the human sciences is likely to be derived from the concept of entropy and the Second Law of Thermodynamics rather than from energy and the First Law (180). The present discussion therefore focuses upon the contrast between a system of theories and actions derived from the conservation of energy and a system derived from entropy considerations.

We start from two sorts of contrast:

First, physical energy is indestructible. Negative entropy (or order) can be, and is, continually created by purposive entities and destroyed by them—or by "random" intrusive events.

Second, energy is a "substance" whose quantity and species are independent of the purposes or state of mind of any organism—there is just so much energy present in a given physical system regardless of our wishes or information. Negative entropy, on the other hand, is a quantity synonymous with information and therefore is determined, at least in part, by the state of mind existing in some human being or other purposive entity. Entropy is a statement of relationship between a purposive entity and some set of objects and events.

These two differences combine to create a profound contrast between those philosophies which emphasize energy alone and those which emphasize entropy in addition to energy. This contrast can be crudely stated by saying that if we rigorously restrict ourselves to seeing man only in terms of energy conservation, our picture of his situation will resemble that of a billiard ball, the prototype of fatalistic nineteenth-century materialism. When, however, we add to energy conservation—for man obeys the

First Law—the idea of entropy, our picture of man becomes a Maxwell's demon, able within wide limits to sort the cards in the pack and to impose his order upon the universe in which he lives—this order being his definition of negative entropy. Such a man could conceivably sort out the isotopes of uranium to control energy sources far beyond those of his own metabolism, or he could paint pictures and set in order the sounds of music for his own enjoyment. He is, it is true, still limited in what he can do. He cannot create perpetual-motion machines, and he is unlikely to be able to break the bank at Monte Carlo. But within the limitations set by his own ignorance (in gambling he deliberately increases his own ignorance by shuffling the cards) and by the conservation of energy and matter and by the fact that he has but limited power to change his own wishes and purposes, the man in this second picture has the freedoms and failings of a human being. He is not passive, but a participant in his own universe.

Now, the billiard-ball picture of man is not a fair representation of the Freudian philosophy of life. In other words, the Freudian theories do not rigorously restrict themselves to seeing man in terms of energy conservation—and, indeed, why should they?

Actually there are at least three lines of thought which change what would be the intolerably limited picture of a billiard ball into something approaching a picture of humanity.

First, psychic energy is linked or equated with motivation, and therefore notions more appropriate to the discussion of entropy and purpose are introduced under cover of this misnomer.

Second, the concept of energy transformation, borrowed from physics, is blurred to give an idea that man can bargain in his energy exchanges.

Third, a series of entelechies (i.e., internal mythical purposive entities or Maxwell's demons)—the id, the ego, the superego (and the animus and anima of Jungian theory)—are introduced into the theoretical system and more or less personified.

Of these three methods of humanizing the picture, the first two are strictly fallacious, but the reasons for humanizing the theoretical picture of man were still good reasons. The only metapsychology which could legitimately be constructed from what Freud knew of the physics of the nineteenth century would have been utterly destructive of the human spirit, and what he produced, while scientifically shaky, was at least less destructive.

Strangely, though Freud has been repeatedly criticized for introducing entelechies into his theoretical system, this seems today to have been a relatively good temporary solution of the problem of purpose which was not then solvable in a more final way. Freud's solution was good in the sense that it is today rather easy to translate these entelechies into more modern concepts. That the human body contains numerous interdependent and self-corrective circuits we now know, and we know the general nature of such circuits. It is therefore easy to imagine in place of such entities as id, ego, and superego, other more complex self-maximating and self-corrective networks. With Freud's energy metaphors, however, nothing can be done except an almost total reconstruction of the theory, starting again from entropy considerations.

Here, however, we are concerned only with the implications of the energy theories for epistemology. We ask only how these theories, right or wrong, have contributed to shape the psychiatrist's view of man.

One verbatim statement from an orthodox Freudian will illustrate what seems to be a general attitude. The speaker was setting up a criterion to distinguish between "magic healing" and "rational treatment," and he derived this criterion from the following proposition, which he treated as a basic postulate: "You cannot achieve a goal without an appropriate expenditure of energy."

Such a postulate determines a whole view of life, and it is worth while to examine its deutero-implications with some care. To begin with, the postulate is a statement of price, with all the possible moral and economic overtones of that concept, including the notions of thrift and waste, and the notion that the expenditure of energy is not in itself pleasant. Further, from the notion of measurable price it is inevitable for the theorist to go on to a grotesque reciprocal quantification not only of "energy" but also of the value of those goals which are to be achieved by the appropriate expenditure. We thus arrive at a philosophy of life and a criterion of health which would derive from measurable "productivity" instead of "creativity." We end with a picture of economic man at his crudest.

It is worth mentioning also that beginning with the crude quantification and economics of "energy," the theorists naturally go on to quantify other related entities. For example: "The patient must first establish positive transference, and that positive transference is gradually used up by the operations of the analyst."

But it may be urged that these quantitative pictures are true and inevitable, and we can only reply that we believe it to be a deutero-picture whose validity is largely a function of man's belief in it; and that such a belief is not necessary can be demonstrated with other quotations. There is, for example, the French proverb *"Pour faire des omelettes, il faut casser des oeufs"* ("You can't make omelets without breaking eggs."). This, in its implications, is quite different from the psychoanalyst's postulate, and is much more closely related to entropy considerations. The French proverb implies that patterns are destroyed in order that other patterns may be created; and the moment price is stated in terms of patterns of this kind, crude quantitative notions of value fly out of the window. Man must still make choices, and to choose A will often mean the destruction or loss of B—but in a world of patterns there can be no common denominator, no simple measure of value. There can be no psychic economics, parallel to the commercial economic theories of the nineteenth century.

As to the general validity of such theories of psychic economics, we would agree that such views of the world can be imposed upon people by the social matrix in which they live, and that people will, at least in part, deutero-learn to see their world in these terms. This, however, is no reason for believing that the theories have more than a deutero-validity. It is not likely that man differs from other animals in having such a grossly simplified system of spiritual values.

Finally, it is necessary to add that while the energy theories occupy such a central position in Freudian theory that Freudians will appeal to them as postulates, there are many more peripheral matters upon which the most orthodox are willing to speak in terms which imply entropy ideas. In the very same lecture on "magical healing" and "rational treatment" from which the sentence about energy was quoted above, the lecturer discussed the effects of diagnosis. His words are worth repeating: "Diagnosis . . . a seeing through the symptoms to the real nature of the disease. . . . It is the province and obligation of the physician to diagnose. . . . It is basically for diagnosis that the patient comes to the doctor, and once diagnosis is made, the doctor is relatively inactive. . . . Cure depends on the patient's willingness to meet the demands of reality as stated in the diagnosis."

In this, as in every statement of insight therapy, there is the premise that the effectiveness of therapy derives not from energy, forces, and the like, but from communication. That which is communicated is called "diagnosis," and this term no doubt includes a vast variety of information at many levels of abstraction, especially information about what we here call the patient's and the therapist's systems of codification. Therapy is thus said to depend in part upon an increase in information (i.e., negative entropy).

Thus the Freudian position—and the position of non-Freudian therapists has been deeply influenced by the Freudians—may be summed up as a mixture of energy phrasings derived consciously from nineteenth-century physics and from phrasings in which entropy ideas are implicit, though not consciously derived from the Second Law of Thermodynamics.

PSYCHIATRY AS A REFLEXIVE SCIENCE

In physics and to some extent in anthropology and other sciences, among them especially history (42), it is now realized that the observer and even the theorist must be included within the systems discussed. The theories of physics and the pronouncements of the historian are alike human constructions and can only be understood as products of an interaction between the data and the human scientist, living in a given epoch in a given culture. The question here discussed is whether psychiatry is today a reflexive science in the sense that psychiatrists habitually regard their theories and practices as human utterance and therefore material for psychiatric study.

Many of the statements of psychiatrists which have been quoted in this chapter demonstrate that the speakers are increasingly studying their own theories and operations from a psychiatric point of view. Four statements may, however, be quoted here to illustrate different sorts of reflexive thinking:

A Jungian: "People do orient themselves to his (Jung's) work through their natural cultural archetype (religious, aesthetic, philosophical, or social). But the Jungian analyst is one who should have worked through that to a truly psychological position . . . which subjects all these to the psychological understanding. . . . It would be regressive from my point of view to fall back upon a religious or philosophical *Weltanschauung.*"

A Freudian: "Metapsychology (is) the coordination of the various points of view (dynamic, historical, and economic)."

A medical psychiatrist: "The first duty of the therapist is to achieve ease. If he himself is anxious or tense, he cannot do therapy. And this is true even if he controls his anxiety. . . . On the whole it is better, if he is anxious, that he should *not* control his anxiety."

A Jungian: "An analysis is a personal relationship within an impersonal framework."

The matter of reflexivity is treated last on the list of items in psychiatric epistemology because it is in regard to this question that the trends and changes of the current psychiatric scene are most evident. Perhaps the greatest contrast between the psychiatric theories of yesterday and the probable psychiatric theories of tomorrow will lie in the degree to which theorists see their own constructions as material for psychiatric study.

The non-reflexive nature of earlier psychoanalytic theory can be illustrated by the statement of a European scholar lecturing on the history of Freudian ideas. He stated, approximately, that Freud thought of psychoanalysis as a historical investigation —especially as an investigation of the analysand's life history. As Freud saw it, the analyst at the end of analysis would have achieved a total survey of relevant and important elements in the life history of the patient from birth up to the moment when that patient entered analysis. In discussion, after the lecture, the lecturer insisted again that the period of life history as studied by Freud terminated at this moment and not at the end of the analysis; and he agreed, speaking as a sophisticated analyst at the present time looking back at the history, that the development of therapeutic theory might have proceeded much faster if Freud had seen the analysis itself as a part of the period under investigation. The lecturer was himself aware of the necessity for reflexiveness in psychiatry, and he was aware that Freud took a different view. Psychoanalysis has always emphasized its close relation to history, and it is therefore interesting to find so dramatic a statement of the non-reflexive nature of early psychoanalytic thinking, when today it is history above all other sciences that has become aware of its own reflexiveness.

The matter is not simple, because, while Freud—at least in the early days—may have taken a non-reflexive position, today some awareness of the reflexive nature of the science of psychiatry is almost if not quite orthodox, and as a result of this change, the whole epistemology of psychiatry is taking on a very different shape. Even in Freud's time it was early realized that the neurotic tendencies of the analyst constituted an important set of factors determining the progress of any analysis, and this, after all, is a first step toward realizing reflexiveness. From early days the analyst has himself been expected, in orthodox circles, to undergo the experience of a training analysis, and among the more thoughtful analysts there is an acceptance of the notion or feeling that this training experience is never completed. For them, the experiences of therapy, in which they now play the role of therapist, are a central part of the ongoing and progressive process of their own lives in which they themselves are achieving or undergoing change. Of these changes they strive to be aware, and therefore they arrive at a reflexive awareness of the therapeutic processes in which they are not only manipulators but participants—both active and passive. For those analysts who see themselves as masters of a craft which they are not concerned to improve but only to use as a means of useful and lucrative employment, this will not be the case; but there exists a leavening of others who see the analytic profession as a continual self-investigation and for whom, therefore, the actual analytic session must always be a reflexive business. To these, therapy is likely to appear not as a goal which can be completed but rather as an ongoing habit of life, acquired in training analysis but continued throughout their professional career.

It would seem to follow that whether the psychiatrist regards psychiatry as a reflexive science or not will determine or be determined by very deep matters in the ethics and practice of his business. His relationship to the patient, his view of human interaction, and his need to defend himself from the patient's attacks will be different according as his pride is invested in a static image of himself as a professional man trained in a certain craft, or in a dynamic image of himself as continually evolving and growing. To the static therapist the uncovering of any mistakes he may make will be a threat; to the dynamic, the discovery of error carries the promise of further advance.

In discussing psychiatry as a branch of pathology it was stated that there is a deep cleavage between those who look for limited goals and those who look for the maintenance of ongoing patterns. Here, in regard to the matter of reflexivity, we have a corresponding contrast between those who are prepared to see therapeutic processes as a one-way causation in which the therapist himself remains essentially unchanged, and those for whom the therapeutic process involves an ongoing dynamic process within the therapist himself. And strangely it is the latter who are, on the whole, in step with the more modern epistemological theories current in the other sciences.

10 · THE CONVERGENCE OF SCIENCE AND PSYCHIATRY

By Gregory Bateson

ALL THAT has been said in the previous chapter about psychiatrists and their culture or habits of thought has been in a sense static. That is, it has been stated that psychiatrists hold certain ideas about energy, about coercion and control, success, normality, and so on; and these ideas have been described as interrelated in a structured system. But the element of time and change has been disregarded. The immediate task is to draw these remarks about psychiatric thinking together into a statement of over-all change.

The thesis of the present chapter is that a large number of piecemeal changes are occurring in psychiatric ways of thought, and that these various changes are interrelated so that, in sum, it is possible to recognize a vast but vaguely defined trend. Further, it will be argued that this trend is related to fundamental changes which are occurring in the more rigorous scientific and philosophical systems of the present day. In fact, there appears to be a convergence between psychiatry and the mathematical, natural, and engineering sciences. Many of those who are contributing to these changes—whether as natural scientists or as psychiatric theorists—feel that there is a deep gulf between the two camps, but it will here be argued that in spite of this deep estrangement a convergence is in process and that this convergence is due to the fact that theorists in both camps are confronting the phenomena of communication and interaction.

257

The first difficulty in assessing change is that the writer is obviously not in a position to say with authority which tendencies are going to win in the current evolution of opinion. The ideas put forward in this book are competing with the others for survival, and we, who are entered in the race, are in no position to predict which horse will win. Moreover, we are only human and therefore will inevitably predict that our own theoretical position is that toward which American psychiatric thinking will evolve.

On the other hand, there are data which we can examine with a somewhat less partisan eye. For example, we can inquire what are the elements in psychiatric thinking against which psychiatrists seem currently to protest. It is impossible for us to jump ahead of the game and to tell in which direction the new ideas and new systems will develop, but it is possible to look at what ideas the psychiatrists are discarding. The next best thing to a statement of the direction in which they are going is a statement about what they are going away from.

It must be remembered that people in general—and psychiatrists are no exception—are necessarily much less articulate about the new thinking toward which they strive than about the old ideas which they would slough away.

We therefore offer a list (Tables A, B, and C) of items against which many psychiatrists currently protest, and in an attempt to predict the future we mention beside each item on this list a contrasting notion to indicate a direction in which evolution is possibly tending. We insist, however, that the list of items from which psychiatric thought is moving away is likely to be more correct than the list of positive directions which, after all, is partly a deduction from the first. The table is, in sum, a list of important controversial foci in the psychiatric field, arranged in the form of polarities. In regard to each controversial matter, the newer ideas are listed in the right-hand column, so that this column constitutes our guess as to the direction in which the general climate of opinion is changing. (We would not, however, lightly discard the possibility of some Hegelian synthesis between the new ideas and the old.)

The mere experience of compiling such a list is sufficient to

TABLE A

Changes in Psychiatric Thought Characterized by Progressively Larger Gestalten

Views away from which psychiatric thought is tending	Views toward which psychiatric thought is tending
Focus upon small Gestalten	Focus upon larger Gestalten
Focus upon structural or synchronic statement	Focus upon process and diachronic statement. The Gestalt studied is enlarged by inclusion of the time dimension
Focus upon parts	Focus upon wholes (64)
Focus upon organs and organ systems in both diagnosis and therapy	Focus upon the organism as a whole as in psychosomatic medicine
Focus determined by the notion that various approaches and disciplines are mutually exclusive (e.g., "organic" versus "functional," etc.)	Focus modified by interdisciplinary and combined approaches
Focus upon the individual	Focus upon interaction
Focus upon systems outside the observer	Focus upon systems in which the observer is included (22), (25), (113), (120), etc.
Focus which omits the social matrix	Focus stresses the social matrix and culture
Focus which sees theories as "objective"	Reflexive focus. The Gestalt is enlarged by including not only the observer but also the theorist and his cultural and psychological bias (15), (42), (43), (130), (131).
Striving for absolutist theories	Striving limited to construction of relativistic theories

TABLE B

Changes Which Are Specially Related to Advances in Scientific Method, Formal Philosophy, and Communications Engineering

Views away from which psychiatric thought is tending	*Views toward which psychiatric thought is tending*
Explanation in terms of Aristotelian "substances"	Description in terms of Galilean variables, as defined by Lewin (97)
Loose additive and subtractive manipulation of "substances" and explanatory variables—often regardless of the Rule of Dimensions	Formal manipulation of variables by multiplication and more complex operations
Attempts to "isolate" variables	Attempts to recognize *constellations* of interdependent variables. At this stage, the engineer's and Gestalt psychologist's ways of thought begin to converge
Emphasis upon quantitative variables	Emphasis upon propositional variables, patterns, and causal networks
Emphasis upon First Law of Thermodynamics and energy economics	Emphasis upon Second Law of Thermodynamics and negative entropy, which is equated with "information"
Study of closed energy systems	Study of open energy systems—e.g., relays, cells, organisms, and patterned aggregates of such systems (28)
Study of lineal causal chains	Study of circular and reticulate causal chains, within which the lineal groupings are seen as only arcs of larger circuits
The search for closed logical systems	The discovery that no such systems can be constructed without contradiction (63)

TABLE C

Changes Which Are Specially Related to the Humanistic Protest

Views away from which psychiatric thought is tending	*Views toward which psychiatric thought is tending*
Valuation of and search for controls, formulae, methods of planned manipulation, coercion, etc.	Valuation of spontaneity, unplanned interaction, etc.
Explanations in terms of causal determinism	Preference for philosophical indeterminism, etc.
Attempts to set up closed systems of explanation	Fear of all cut-and-dried systems, which are viewed as "mechanistic"

demonstrate that the changes cannot really be regarded as separable items. If the reader doubts this, he is invited to compile his own list of the foci of change. He will find that some more abstract bridge exists between every pair of items in his list and therefore that he is forced to adopt some classification of the items. Further, he will find that many alternative classifications are possible because the items are parts of a complex interlinked whole.

One way of roughly classifying these interrelated items is illustrated in the tables. In Table A are listed those changes which appear to be increases in the Gestalt studied. Table B lists those trends which are specifically related to the formal discoveries of those philosophers, mathematicians, and engineers who have dealt with problems of communication. Table C lists trends which we describe as "humanistic"—i.e., foci of controversy in which the newer ideas appear to be a protest against the reduction of the human individual to materialistic or crude biological terms.

Undoubtedly all of these listed items are parts of a general revolt against nineteenth-century scientism with its ideas of simplicity, control, manipulation, formulae, and the like. Further, it seems that this revolt is occurring both among humanists and among those formal scientists and philosophers who are concerned with the problems of communication.

It seems that for all items of Table A, which lists the various increases in the size of the Gestalt, both the humanists and the engineers will be in agreement on the direction in which they believe a change of thinking is desirable.

Increase in size and scope of the Gestalt is desired by the humanists because it gives a sense of freedom: data which are cut and dried and depersonalized when seen as elements in a small Gestalt take on an appearance of life, vitality, and freedom when seen as elements in larger wholes. Even with extreme extension of the Gestalt to include the whole perceptual universe, the thinker can envisage a mystical monism and can identify himself as a living part of an almost living whole.

For entirely different reasons, the formal scientist is driven also to prefer the larger Gestalten. He does not seek these by preference (unless he himself has leanings toward the mystical), because his whole professional bias is toward reducing Gestalten to the smallest complexity which will afford him what he regards as sufficient insight. His training in the use of the rule of parsimony and Ockham's razor predisposes him to keep the Gestalten small. But, when he has proved to himself, against his own professional preference, that it is necessary to think in terms of larger and more complex units, he will insist upon this necessity. The doctrine of the larger Gestalt must first be forced upon him by his findings, but thenceforward he and the humanist will share the preference for large Gestalten. The engineer or scientist will insist upon these large Gestalten because he values clarity and completeness of explanation; the humanist because he values life and its complexities.

It is a strange convergence that is occurring, and one which makes strange bedfellows. Nineteenth-century scientism was apparently the stimulus for two movements: That of the humanists occurred outside the subculture of the professional natural scientists and was a protest against the cut-and-dried causal formulae of the natural scientists of the previous generation. The other movement—that of the formal scientists—occurred within the subculture of the natural sciences, where it was a move forced upon the scientists by their data. The physicist found that he could understand his data only when he realized that they were collected by his own activities interfering in some degree with the external world which he was attempting to study. Therefore he was compelled to include the observer within the system studied. Similarly he found that he could understand his own ideas only when he accepted the fact that they were his, and therefore in part determined by the culture and epoch in which he was living. Thenceforward he was forced to accept the reflexive nature of his theoretical constructions—i.e., to include the theorist as well as the observer within the system studied.

The change toward larger Gestalten and the necessity of this change for both humanistic and formal reasons can be illustrated by considering Sullivan's emphasis (120), (160) upon the phenomena of interaction. This emphasis is very clearly part of a defense of man against the older, more mechanistic thinking which saw him so heavily determined by his internal psychological structure that he could easily be manipulated by pressing the appropriate buttons—a doctrine which made the therapeutic interview into a one-way process, with the patient in a relatively passive role. The Sullivanian doctrine places the therapeutic interview on a human level, defining it as a significant meeting between two human beings. The role of the therapist is no longer to be dehumanized in terms of definable purposes which he can plan, and the role of the patient is no longer dehumanized into that of an object of manipulation. The Sullivanian emphasis upon interaction is thus a metacommunicative statement of the value to be set upon man and upon human relations. It is a humanistic correction of older manipulative emphases.

If, on the other hand, we look at the same Sullivanian doctrine of interaction with the eyes of a mathematician or circuit engineer, we find it to be precisely the theory which emerges as appropriate when we proceed from the fact that the two-person system has circularity (147). From the formal, circularistic point of view no such interactive system can be totally determined by any one of its parts: neither person can effectively manipulate the other. In fact, not only humanism but also rigorous communications theory leads to the same conclusion: that the problems are those of interaction as well as of internal structure. If therapy is a matter of correcting false or idiosyncratic codification, we arrive again at an emphasis upon interaction but get there by way of formal communications theory rather than by way of the recognition that man is "human."

Another example which illustrates how the humanistic and circularistic approaches partially coincide in what they attempt to say is to be derived from the contrast between Jungian and Freudian attitudes toward the unconscious components of the personality. The Freudian attitude may be summed up in terms of the famous dictum, "Where id is, there ego shall be." The Jungian position is vague but seems to be an insistence that the fullness of life depends upon accepting the fact that most of the individual's mental processes are of necessity unconscious and that he must live with them. Both schools alike start from recognition of the unconscious and from the assumption that in the mental life of the patient before therapy, the unconscious components are foreign bodies in the stream of psychic life. The Freudian ambition to substitute ego for id or to include the id within the scope of the ego, sounds to Jungians like advocating manipulative and conscious control of the foreign body. In reply to this they would urge merely the acceptance —even the joyful acceptance—of the fact that the foreign body though always and inevitably unconscious is really a part of the self and the self a part of it—the collective unconscious being imagined to be in some sense greater than the self.

In this contrast between the two schools in their evaluation of the unconscious, it appears that the Jungian is less articulate, more mystical, and at the same time more humanistic, while the Freudian at first sight appears to be the more articulate, scientific, and materialistic. In caricature, we might describe the Freudians as cold, objective, and even pragmatic, while the Jungians in analogous caricature would appear to be dewy-eyed nature boys, all sweetness and light (and this is approximately how the Freudians see them).

When, however, the question of the status of unconscious processes is posed in engineering terms, it appears that the formal statement about circular systems will be in step with the Jungian rather than the Freudian position. The engineers, it is true, will not exhibit dreamy-eyed enthusiasm (with the possible exception of the Dianeticians), but they will tell us very simply that no part of a circular or reticulate system can be governed by or included within another part because the parts of the system are themselves interactive. They will regard Freud's dictum as itself a dream, and in reply to any ambitious dream of increasing the scope either of the ego or of unconsciousness, they might use the iceberg as a crude analogy. The proportion of an iceberg which is visible above the level of the sea cannot be increased by adding more ice to the top. Similarly, about consciousness the engineers will say that if this phenomenon is to be thought of as the function of some part of the mental apparatus in which reports from other parts are centralized, then the informational content of such a consciousness can always be only a small fraction of the total mental activity. They will argue that for every addition (increment 1) to the apparatus of consciousness, a very much greater further addition (increment 2) will be necessary if the activities of increment 1 are themselves to be made conscious; and that again a still further increment will be necessary if the activities of increment 2 are also to be reported upon to consciousness; and so on.

Moreover, the circularities of Jungian theory, which Jung and others have supported by references to the *mandala* of Tibet and to the Golden Flower of Chinese mysticism—a form of argument which is literary, artistic, mystical, and humanistic rather than rigorous—will fall into place beside the phrasings of communications theory as rather direct—i.e., very slightly symbolical—statements about the processes which must be supposed to occur in intrapersonal and interpersonal communication.

Thus again we reach the curious and unexpected position that though there may be many disputes still unsettled between the formal engineers on the one hand, and the humanists on the other, there is an overlap in what the two groups are attempting to say. Moreover, this overlapping extends even to matters of violent feeling. Among humanistic psychiatrists, the assault upon the psyche which occurs in electric shock therapy and in such operational procedures as lobotomy is seen as gross and potentially destructive. The humanistic attitude toward these procedures may be summarized in a word: horror. But the horror which humanists express is no less than that expressed by the engineers who see in these operations a blind and stupid muddling, a destruction of the organism's precious negative entropy. One of them once remarked bitterly to the writer, "I suppose a lobotomized patient wouldn't mind working on the atom bomb."

From what has been said so far, it might appear that we could examine any given individual as to his opinions and ways of thought and form a quantitative judgment as to his position between the two extreme poles of nineteenth-century scientism on the one hand and interactive communication theory on the other. But, in fact, this is impossible. If we attempt such a diagnosis of individual scientists, what we find is that each individual has a very complex gamut of views so that he will express views in one area which would place him as ahead of the general climate of opinion (e.g., in seeing the therapeutic process as an interaction) while in another area he will cling to characteristically nineteenth-century positions (e.g., in regard to the economics of psychic energy).

It must be remembered, after all, that the newer position, as a whole, is uncrystallized and that in their extreme form the newer ideas would seem to threaten the very basis of communication, reducing all the world to a Heraclitean flux. It is therefore common to find that a person has his fixed points of conservatism in regard to which he will make assertions characteristic of nineteenth-century thinking, but if reassured in regard to these fixed points, he will launch out into exploration of less rigid notions in other areas of theory. There is probably no individual or philosophical system which is consistently "modern" in these matters, and this generalization applies both to the "humanists" and to the formal scientists.

Merely to state, however, that the humanists and the formal scientists are alike in looking towards the larger Gestalten and alike in finding that it is difficult or impossible to do this consistently is not enough. It is necessary also to ask whether both the humanist and the formal scientist are in fact extending the Gestalten in the same ways and dimensions. This question can be examined by means of an example.

Let us imagine four persons in a wood: first, a woodman with an ax cutting a tree, himself skilled but with his thoughts unencumbered by the complexities of epistemological and scientific probing; second, a nineteenth-century scientist; third, a humanist—perhaps an artist or a poet; and fourth, a scientist of the more modern circularistic variety. Now let us consider for a moment what the three professional thinkers can contribute to a knowledge or understanding of the woodman's activity. The nineteenth-century scientist will contribute formulae for the penetration of a simplified fictitious ax blade of mass M, moving at velocity V, and striking a fictitious homogeneous substance of viscosity v; etc. He will give us the trajectories of fictitious (perhaps spherical) chips flying in a simplified atmosphere. He may even give us formulae linking together some of the variables in the woodman's muscular activity. And so on. He will say very little about himself—except to imply by his very reticence that he is unwilling to look at that self.

The humanist, on the other hand, be he artist or poet, will tell us much about himself. He may even include the observer within the system studied to such an extent that he excludes the woodman and the scene in the wood. In an extreme (but not rare) example, the humanist might be obscurely touched by the resolved contrast between strength and precision in the woodman's movements; and this resolution of contrast, felt rather than consciously perceived, might shape some musical or other abstract form, in the creation of which the artist's strength and precision will also themselves be exerted and combined: the contrast will thus be resolved simultaneously on two levels.

In such a case, the created object—the poem, the painting, or the music—will carry important deutero-messages. It may enrich the experience of the persons whose life it touches because these deutero-messages are somehow forged into the created thing. The artist will have said something obscurely true of a number of relationships—of the relationship between the woodman and his ax, of the relationship between himself and the woodman, of the relationship between himself and his instrument or medium, and of the relationship between himself and his audience. The humanistic insistence that the Gestalt be extended to include the observer leads thus to the making of statements which are relevant to the human spirit. But the humanist—be he artist or even poet—will be unable to say what it is that he has said.

The circularistic scientist, on the other hand, will start where his nineteenth-century predecessor left off; he will accept the formulae describing the penetration of the ax and the flying of the chips and the muscular activity of the woodman, and he will go on from these formulae to attempt a fuller picture. He will discover, for example, that, quite apart from anything contained in these formulae, the strokes of the ax form a complex series, each single stroke being partially determined by the state of the tree trunk left by the previous strokes. The examination of this series will lead him into very difficult problems which he cannot dismiss as, even in principle, solved by the nineteenth-century formulae. As he examines these problems he will be forced to include the characteristics and especially the purposive characteristics of the woodman in his description. Among these characteristics there will be such items as the relationship between strength and precision, together with many others which might also have affected the humanist or artist.

At this point, the resemblance between the formal scientist and the humanist might seem to be maximal, thenceforward to diminish. But, while it is true that what the scientist will make of the relation between precision and strength is not at all like the artist's synthesis, the contrast will not be as great as might be expected, because the scientist is himself a human being and is aware of this fact as a relevant piece of the system which he is trying to describe. His study will branch out as a study of the interactive relationships present in the system, and his synthesis will contain many levels of reference. When he discusses the combination of strength and precision, not only will he see in this combination the crude engineering problem of combining great forces with microscopic self-correction but also he will see the recurrence of this problem in his own activities as an observer and analyst.

Without the knowledge that he himself is a human organism, the scientist's formulae, like those of the nineteenth-century scientist discussed above, would cut across the fabric of life, regardless of that weft and structure which other living organisms have slowly built up in their search for codification and negative entropy. He might, for example, assert that people are entirely understandable when seen as self-maximating economic entities—an assertion which would cut across all the complexities of human relationship and which might lead to great pathology should people attempt to live that way. But with the knowledge of his own humanity, the scientist has the possibility of groping forward toward a synthesis which shall not affront the artist.

One difference, however, will remain: the scientist will always set a special value upon knowing just what it is that he is saying. The artist may be content when he is sure that his creation rings true against the touchstone of his own emotional integrity; the scientist must also examine the internal logic of his synthesis and test it against later observations. To do this, the scientist must be clear about what it is that he is saying. His hypothesis, like the artist's creation, is a codification of data; and if he is to test this hypothesis, he must be aware of his own processes of codification. He must know the operations by which external events were recorded—i.e., codified—to provide data; and he must know how these data were manipulated and transformed (recodified) to become hypotheses. To be aware of what he is saying, the scientist must know his own system of codification; the artist or humanist need not make this particular effort.

A contrast therefore still remains. No doubt much of the horror which humanists express vis-à-vis the scientist is due to misunderstanding: either the scientist is obsolete in his clinging to nineteenth-century crudities or the humanist is behind the times in his understanding of current scientific approaches. But still an element in the humanist's horror is due to a real difference between the humanistic and even the most sophisticated scientific approaches. This difference must be examined, and at this point it is convenient to turn from generalities drawn from our discussion of the imagined scene in the wood to the more specific problems of culture and psychiatric theory.

Psychiatry—and this includes not only theories but also the operations and ethics of the therapist—is apparently evolving slowly in two directions, one which we call humanistic and one which we call circularistic, for lack of a better term. A broad area in which these two trends overlap has been described, but one significant difference has emerged—namely, in the degree of articulacy which the psychiatrist should attempt. If he favors the humanistic trend, the psychiatrist will be content with a rather slight understanding of the operational steps and codification of his own thought. He will then test the validity of his synthesis and of his therapeutic operations as an artist might, against his own emotional integrity. If, on the other hand, he is a circularist, he will strive for total articulacy and test his synthesis by the criteria of logical coherence and factual prediction. Moreover, this contrast defines a dilemma which is real in the sense that each of the conflicting views offers certain advantages which must be lost by a too close adherence to the opposing view. The humanist will surely have the advantage in the actual therapeutic session because he is free to respond swiftly and smoothly as a human being facing his patient in shared humanity. He is—like the woodman or the artist— unencumbered by the load of analytic procedures and computations which must weigh down the circularist. The humanist, like the artist, can act spontaneously out of his own integrity and need not always stop to determine exactly what he is saying.

On the other hand, the humanist will never create a cumulative science, for he cannot clearly transmit his wisdom to his successors. In so far as psychiatry remains an art it will build up no body of growing and testable hypotheses. In an art, the conventions and fashions change from epoch to epoch, and the deutero-messages which the artist communicates change with the times. But art is not an appropriate medium for the study of the nature of such messages because the artist must always leave his own systems of codification implicit and unexamined.

The precise and even compulsive examination of such systems is the task of the scientist; and he, by this very compulsiveness and precision, is rendered clumsy and bereft of the grace and easy movement in interaction which, to be a skillful therapist, he would need. He may spend years building up the mathematical formulae describing interaction; but the humanist may learn more about how to interact by spending a few hours on a dance floor.

Gradually, no doubt, compromises will be found. The formulating scientists will build up methods of describing with increasing precision what occurs in a therapeutic session between humanist and patient. Some part of this precise description will gradually be absorbed by the humanists, who will thereby become able to improve their methods. They will then alter the character of the therapeutic session, and the scientist must then start again to describe it. The whole process of advance in theory and practice in a human science is like a strange variant of the famous race between Achilles and the tortoise. Every significant hypothesis which the theorist creates from his observations of the practitioner contributes to the inarticulate and mobile skills of the latter, enabling him again to forge ahead of the theorist, who must now make new observations.

But perhaps more important than this agreement about their respective roles—and the compromise suggested above really consists in an assignment of roles—is one feature of the formal scientist's epistemology which has not yet been mentioned in this chapter. Central to the fear and dislike which the humanists express when they meet with the formulae of the scientists is the idea that the latter will assert that some hypothesis is final and complete. The humanist believes that any such final and comprehensive statement would be the destruction of his value system and would finally and irreversibly reduce the patient to an object of manipulation. It would surely do so—but the scientist today knows that no such hypothesis can be constructed without leading to contradiction or to infinite retrogression. Goedel's discovery (63) that no system of propositions can be complete in itself and not lead to contradiction may be interpreted to mean that Achilles can never catch the tortoise in the race which we are discussing. The theorist can only build his theories about what the practitioner was doing yesterday. Tomorrow the practitioner will be doing something different because of these very theories.

11 · INDIVIDUAL, GROUP, AND CUL-TURE: A Review of the Theory of Human Communication

By Jurgen Ruesch and Gregory Bateson

SCIENTIFIC theory traditionally distinguishes between that which is assumed to exist in reality and that which is actually perceived by a human observer. The difference in the picture between assumed reality and perceived reality is explained as being due to the peculiarities and limitations of the human observer. In the study of human communication, it is difficult if not impossible to distinguish between assumed and perceived reality. As psychiatrists and social scientists we are, by definition, interested to inquire into the ways an observer perceives the world rather than how this world really is, because the only method we possess to infer the existence of the real world is to compare one observer's views with the views of other observers. Discrepancies in these views then permit us to make some inferences about the psychological processes of the observers, and by combining the various observations to gain a picture of what one might call assumed reality. Whether this assumed reality is a true picture of what really happens, nobody is in a position to decide.

None the less, the assumption of "reality" is usually helpful. The closest approximation to what the physicist calls "reality" can be obtained, in the field of communication, by assuming that a superhuman observer looks at human communication from a position outside of the social systems which he studies, so that he, as an observer, is unlikely to influence the phenomena he is going to observe. The picture which he might obtain from such a vantage point is sketched in Figure 4 and described in detail in Table D. In constructing such an outline, the assumption is made that a human observer can focus upon various aspects of communication, with various magnifications, while the limitations and characteristics of his perceptual apparatus remain the same. The analogy that can be referred to at this point is the field of vision seen when looking through a microscope. Depending upon the magnification used, the structure of the objects studied in the field will appear in smaller or greater detail, and as magnification increases, the area of the field must decrease. Similarly the human observer, when looking at communication, can have only one focus at any one time. Depending upon whether he focuses upon small or large entities, he will see the various functions in greater or smaller detail. It follows that the processes of receiving, evaluating, and transmitting can be observed at the intrapersonal, interpersonal, group, and cultural levels of organization. In Figure 4, the various processes of communication have been represented by sectors of a cone. At the intrapersonal level, the focus of the observer is limited by the self, and the various functions of communication are found within the self. At the interpersonal level the perceptual field is occupied by two people, at the group level by many people, and at the cultural level by many groups. Concomitantly, in each of these fields, the importance of the single individual diminishes, and at the higher levels one person becomes only a small element in the system of communication.

The focus of the human observer is not fixed; rather it has to be viewed as a fluctuating or oscillating phenomenon in which quick glances are taken rapidly at various levels and at various functions. Communication is an extremely dynamic phenomenon with a rapid rate of change of levels and of functions, which range from evaluation to transmission and conduction.

Matters are relatively simple if we assume the existence of an observer looking from outside at our human communication

THE LEVELS OF COMMUNICATION

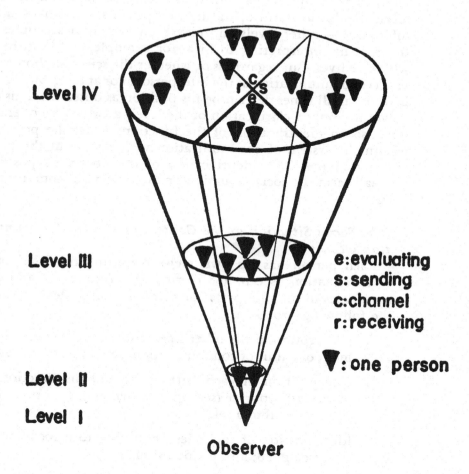

Level IV

Level III

e: evaluating
s: sending
c: channel
r: receiving

▼: one person

Level II

Level I

Observer

systems. Matters become more complicated if we introduce a human observer who himself is an integral part of the system. For psychiatric purposes, the observer can be assumed to operate at the interpersonal level, and hence we shall discuss matters of communication as pertaining to an observer who operates at this level. In other words, the observer, who in this case happens to be the psychiatrist, explores the examinee's communication system at the interpersonal level and makes inferences as to the events which take place at the intrapersonal level. In addition, still operating interpersonally, he may make inferences at other levels and may even communicate these to the patient, interpreting to him, for example, the culture in which he lives. But regardless of whether the scientist chooses to observe communication at the interpersonal or at the group level, he must at all times determine his position as observer. This involves not only a clarification of the levels at which he operates but also an identification of the functions which he possesses within the system of communication which he is in the process of studying. The identification of the observer's position we shall term the social situation or the context of communication.

I. The Social Situation or the Context in Which Communication Occurs

Each person has his own views regarding the label of a social situation (see p. 398 in ref. 149). Agreement and discrepancies in the interpretation of the situation depend upon the following processes:

A. "Perception of the other's perception," or the establishment of a unit of communication (see pp. 203, 208, 280).

B. The position of each participant and his function as observing reporter (see pp. 24, 197, 199; also p. 110 in ref. 147; p. 189 in ref. 180).

C. Identification of the rules pertaining to a social situation (see p. 28; also p. 401 in ref. 149).

D. Identification of the roles in a social situation (see p. 27; also p. 405 in ref. 149).

II. The Networks of Communication

All types of network (p. 29) are coexistent, but the relevance of one of these is determined by the participant's pur-

TABLE D

The Specification of Networks at the Four Levels of Communication

LEVELS	ORIGIN OF MESSAGE	SENDER	CHANNELS	RECEIVER	DESTINATION OF MESSAGE
I. Intrapersonal "within one"	Sensory end organ or Communication center.		Neural, humoral pathways and contiguous pathways.	Communication center or the effector organs.	
II. Interpersonal "one to one"	Communication center of person sending message.	Effector organ of sending person.	Sound, light, heat, odor, vibrations traveling across space on the one hand, chemical or mechanical contact with material or person on the other hand.	Sensory end organs of receiving person.	Communication center of person receiving message.
III. A. Group "One to many" (centrifugal messages)	Communication center of group: head man or committee.	Person specializing in being a mouthpiece or executive for the communication center.	Multiplication of message through press, radio, loudspeaker system, movies, circulars, etc.	Persons engaged in receiving and interpreting incoming messages for the group—readers, listeners, theater spectators, critics.	Many persons who are members of a group. Identity of persons is unspecified by name; they are known by role. Group is specified.
B. Group "Many to one" (centripetal messages)	Many persons who are members of a group. Identity of persons is unspecified by name; they are known by role. Group is specified.	Spokesman who expresses the voice of the people, the family, or other small groups at the periphery.	Mail, word of mouth, or other instrumental actions of people.	Professional specialists who engage in receiving messages: news analysts, intelligence service, government agencies. Condensation and abstraction of incoming messages.	Communication center of group—executive, committee, or head man.
IV. A. Cultural "Space binding" messages of "many to many"	Many groups unspecified by name, known by role, which express moral, aesthetic, or religious views—e.g., the clergy, children.	Groups specializing in the formulation of standards of living: legislators.	Script, written and unwritten regulations and laws. Customs transmitted by personal contact often implicit in action. Persons become channel.	Groups engaging in the reception and interpretation of cultural messages such as judges, lawyers, scientists, ministers.	Many groups composed of living people, unspecified by name, known by role.
B. Cultural "Time binding" messages of "many to many"	Many unspecified groups the members of which are older than the receivers or already dead.	The voice of the past, frequently a mythological or historical figure.	Script, material culture such as objects, architectural structures, etc., and personal contact from generation to generation often implicit in action.	Group specializing in the reception and interpretation of the messages of the past—archaeologists, historians, clergy.	Many unspecified groups the members of which are younger than the originators of the message.

277

poses. The observer will focus upon the participant's exchange of messages, and the extent of the network used will determine at which level the observer will have to analyze the events (see p. 7 in ref. 151). The choice of the network also determines the metacommunicative processes (p. 203)—that is, the explicit or implicit instructions of the participants to each other and to the observer as to the way the messages ought to be interpreted.

A. *The intrapersonal network* is characterized by the fact that:

—The self-observer (see p. 199) is always totally participant.

—Both the place of origin and the destination of messages are located within the sphere of one organism (see p. 38); and the correction of errors is therefore difficult, if not impossible (see p. 199).

—The system of codification used can never be examined (see p. 200).

Within the intrapersonal network (see p. 29) three distinct groups of functions can be distinguished:

1. *Reception* includes both proprioception and exteroception. Proprioception gives information about the state of the organism; in popular language these data, if consciously perceived, are referred to as feelings or sensations. In proprioception the end organs are predominantly internal and react to chemical and mechanical stimuli (see p. 30; also p. 22 in ref. 150); in exteroception the end organs are located on or near the surface of the body, and give information about relations between the self and the environment (see p. 197; also p. 23 in ref. 150). The exteroceptive end organs react to wave phenomena, such as light and sound, in addition to other mechanical and chemical stimuli.

2. *Transmission* includes both propriotransmission and exterotransmission (see p. 30). In propriotransmission, nervous impulses travel on the efferent path-

ways to the smooth muscles, and chemical impulses travel along humoral pathways for purposes of regulation of the organism. In exterotransmission the contraction of the striped muscles is used for action upon the outside world, including communication with other individuals (see p. 203).

3. The *central functions* include coordination, interpretation, and storage of information (see pp. 169, 183).

Information received through proprioception or propriotransmission is complementary to information acquired through exteroception or exterotransmission (see pp. 22–23 in ref. 150). The complementary relation between proprioception and exteroception is such that complete information could only be obtained by a combination of these two functions. Such total combination seems, however, to be impossible, and in its functioning the organism seems to specialize at certain moments in one or the other mode of experience, with resulting failure to act upon data which might have been derived from the other mode: pain may preclude external perceptiveness, and exposure to violent external events may preclude awareness of pain or fatigue.

B. *The interpersonal network* is characterized by the fact that:

—The potentialities for receiving, transmitting, and evaluating messages are equally divided and therefore the system consists of potentially equivalent parts, the participating individuals. The directional flow of messages characteristic of the neural network is therefore absent. Both the place of origin and the destination of messages is known to the senders and the recipients; therefore correction of information is possible.

—The person engaged in observation of others must of necessity be partially participating, partially observing. When observing, a bigger Gestalt is considered; when participating, the Gestalt is narrowed in accordance with the individual's purposes. Both participation and observation are parts of experience and therefore means of collecting information. The two types of information so gained complement each other, but the complementation is never complete (see p. 203; also p. 98 in ref. 120; p. 393 in ref. 149). At any one moment the individual must specialize in one or the other of the modes of experience and must therefore fail to collect the information which might have been gathered by the other mode.

From this complementary relation and from the fact that the gathering of complete information is impossible, it follows that the human individual can never perceive himself perfectly in relation to others. There is always a discrepancy between his more proprioceptive view of himself and that knowledge of himself which he gets through his own exteroceptors, or from the observations of others (see pp. 394–396 in ref. 149). Similarly he cannot entertain at the same moment both a proprioceptive picture of himself and a picture of himself as defined by his status or social situation (see p. 408 in ref. 149).

C. The *group network* is characterized by the fact that:
—The potentialities for receiving and transmitting are unequally divided among the persons. This restriction or specialization of function is characteristic of all organization and has the effect of re-establishing in some degree the directional flow of messages. It also unites the individuals into a larger unit capable of carrying out the three great functions of reception, transmission, and coordination.
—Typically, in larger organized groups only the source or only the destination of many messages is distinct and known to the participants; the unknown part is related to the fact that individuals may either act as source and destination, or as channels which merely

relay the message to the other individuals. The correction of messages is therefore delayed and frequently is possible only by short-cutting the traditionally established pathways (see p. 39).

Essentially two types of messages can be distinguished:

1. Communication of "one person to many" constitutes primarily a one-way flow of messages from the center to the periphery. Reply to this flow is delayed, if it occurs at all. The "one" person is more actively engaged in transmission, while the "many" are more concerned with receiving (see p. 38).

2. Communication of "many persons to one" is primarily a one-way flow of messages towards a center. Progressive abstraction of messages is necessary because of the limited capacity of the receiver. The "one" person is more engaged in receiving, while the "many" tend to engage in active transmission (see p. 39).

From what has been said about complementarity, it follows that the completeness of information obtained by any given individual in an organized group decreases with every increase in complexity and differentiation of the system. In the organized groups each individual is assigned specialized functions, either as observer or as transmitter or as coordinator, and this specialization implies impoverished perception. It is conspicuous also that where two groups are in contact, the information upon which the members of each group base their pictures of their own and of the other group is inflexible, stereotyped, and projective (see p. 402 in ref. 149).

D. *The cultural network.* In addition to intrapersonal, interpersonal, and organized group networks, which are variously perceived as such by the individuals, there is a host of instances in which the individual is unable to recognize the source and destination of messages, and therefore does not recognize that these messages travel in a network structure. For lack of a better word we describe this unperceived system as the cultural network, since many of the premises of every culture are carried in this way (see p. 41).

It is characteristic of this network that messages are transmitted from many persons to many. The sources and destination of messages are, however, unknown; the potentialities for receiving and transmitting are unascribed; and the correction of information is therefore impossible (see p. 40).

When participating in a cultural network, people are in many cases unaware of being the receivers or senders of messages. Rather the message seems to be an unstated description of their way of living. They attribute to it no human origin, but they themselves transmit the message to others by living in accordance with its content, which they may regard as "human nature" (see p. 41).

Examples of messages which are commonly carried by such an unperceived network are:

—Messages about language, and linguistic systems (see p. 43).

—Ethical premises (see p. 42; p. 108 in ref. 147).

—Theories of man's relation to the universe and to his fellow man (see p. 42).

In addition to being implicit in the daily life and material culture of the individual, such messages may be carried also by such vehicles as:

—The printed word (see ref. 73; ref. 117): historical and mythological documents and monuments (see p. 43; also p. 108 in ref. 147).

E. *Short circuits in larger networks:* In addition to the well-established channels along which the flow of messages runs, it is common to find short cuts which reduce the time of transmission and diminish the number of intermediary stations. In the case of the large superpersonal networks, interpersonal links are introduced which personalize the mass communication (e.g., the personal

emissaries of government). In intrapersonal or interpersonal networks, the function of the short circuit is
to convey alarm signals (see p. 39) which maintain the
cohesion of that particular network by giving warning of
its threatened dissolution, often with good effect (e.g.,
anxiety) (see p. 37).

III. *Technical Characteristics of Communication*

The technical description of communication includes statements about the communication machinery, the methods of
codifying data, the effect of these data upon the behavior of
the system, and a general theory of the nature of information
(see pp. 168–211).

A. *Statements about codification.* In all communication occurring in networks of different orders, it is necessary to
describe the transformation (codification) whereby data
about events and objects of various kinds come to be
represented by other events (the message) in the network. The present state of knowledge is totally inade-
quate to permit any precise statement as to the technical
nature of internal codification. It has, however, been
suggested that the brain is preponderantly digital in its
functioning and that this digital functioning is elaborated to permit the mental handling of Gestalten.

1. At the intrapersonal level: To describe codification is
to specify the relation between the neural, chemical,
and other signals and the internal or external events
to which they refer (see pp. 168–211, 199).

2. At the interpersonal level, the description of codifica-
cation will define the symbolization processes of language together with the more tenuous symbolisms
present in nonverbal communication (see p. 201).

3. At the group level, in addition to the verbal and nonverbal processes, present at the interpersonal level,
we meet with new types of symbolization not ordinarily regarded as such. The patterns of the organiza-

tion of the group leave traces in the participating individuals. However, inasmuch as these individuals do not act as stations of origin or destination of messages, but often as channels only, codification at this level requires intactness in the organization as a whole. The group in action possesses the information, not the individual (see p. 39).

4. At the cultural level, the codification is again entirely different. At the intrapersonal and interpersonal levels, codification is characteristically atomistic: separable and isolable events, such as the neural impulse or the word symbol, stand for separable events in the outside world. At the group level, there is apparently no such atomism; and the organization of the group is evidence of codification. At the cultural level the organization is beyond the reach of observation of the individual, who implicitly carries the cultural message in his actions of everyday life. Being an infinitesimal part of the network, the individual's function as communication channel is overshadowed by the importance of intrapersonal and interpersonal events (see pp. 40, 44, 221, 225).

B. *Quantitative statements about the functioning network.* These include statements about:

1. *Capacity of receivers,* transmitters, and channels; the actual load of the circuits (overload, jamming, underload) (see p. 106 in ref. 155).

2. *Threshold Problems:* The definition of conditions which must be met for one relay to affect another. Description of changes in such conditions (e.g., due to age, past events, and the impact of hormones, toxins, and other physiological agents) (see p. 259 in ref. 107).

3. *Time characteristics of the relays:* Refractory period, latency, summation characteristics, and the like. These features are relevant at all levels, whether the relays

are neurons or human individuals (see p. 74 in ref. 180).

4. *Statements about upkeep, metabolism, and replacement of parts of the system:* The organizational continuity of the various systems is maintained, but the constituent parts are usually subject to constant replacement. It is therefore necessary to describe the processes by which new parts are assimilated into the organization of the system. This is achieved by study of the organism's energy exchanges, its exploitation of negative entropy in the environment for the maintenance of its own internal negative entropy or organization. Where the constituent parts of the system are human individuals, it is also necessary to examine the processes of exchange of information between persons. Experience of such interaction, being organized, determines in itself the future organization (see ref. 153; p. 20 in ref. 181).

5. *Statements about the stability and adaptability of the system:* These include statements about the variables by which the steady state is defined and a description of the limits of internal change beyond which the system is unable to correct deviations. These two aspects together define the conditions under which irreversible change must occur. Living within these limits can be regarded as the broad purpose of any system (see ref. 37; p. 116 in ref. 147).

C. *The informational state of the system.* At any given moment in the life of a system a large number of its characteristics are determined by previous events. While these learned characteristics are already subsumed in the total description of the network, it is convenient also to regard these features as an aggregate of information. In such special description previous events are referred to as "experience" and the effects of such experience are assumed to be codified messages or signs. It is also possible that many characteristics of the system, determined by genetics rather than by environment, can also conveniently be regarded as information.

For the observer, and even for the self-observer, data about the informational state of an organism can only be obtained by observing its self-corrective activities (see p. 201).

The informational state of larger networks such as the organized group is exceedingly difficult to estimate. However, it is possible to regard the changes in the social network which result from group experience—for example, war—as a kind of information. The seat of this information is not in the individual alone, nor is it contained in stored records, but rather it is found in the changed topology of the social pathways of communication, whereby the group as a whole is enabled to react in a modified way when faced with a repetition of the experience (see p. 181 in ref. 180).

D. *Knowledge and its effect.* Every message is to be regarded as a statement about the past, but every such statement within a self-corrective system necessarily has implications for the future and especially for future action on the part of the recipient. Every message is both indicative and imperative. From the observer's standpoint the indicative characteristics of a message are amplified by study of the system from which it emanates, while its imperative effectiveness is determined by the character of the system upon which it impinges (see p. 179; also p. 96 in ref. 155).

IV. *Interaction and Self-Correction*

The study of interaction is concerned with the effect of communication upon the behavior of the two or more interacting entities. This study therefore always involves making statements at two, if not more, levels of abstraction: there must be statements about the participating entities, and there must also be statements about that larger entity which is brought into being by the fact of interaction. Even in the relationship between a person and a thing, interaction occurs: the person is self-corrective as a result of his observations of the effect which his actions seem to have upon the thing (see ref. 134). Similarly, authoritarian relationships (when one or more participants are treated as "things") can never be fully described as one-way communication. Only when information regarding the effects of action returns to affect the system is self-correction possible.

It follows from this that interaction sequences always and necessarily contain an element of unpredictability for the participants. At a given instant the individual does not yet have the information which he will have later when the effect of his action becomes observable. Any predictions which he may make about his own later actions must therefore contain an element of guesswork. If he is rigidly bound by his own guesses to the extent, for example, of ignoring the later information, the larger system of which he is only a part will be rigid and incapable of self-correction.

The study of interaction thus becomes a study of the success or failure of ongoing self-correction. It is concerned with the ability of an entity to predict events and also with the entity's ability to modify its action when these predictions are shown to be in error (see p. 263; also p. 97 in ref. 155; p. 113 in ref. 180; ref. 160).

A. *Interaction at various levels.* Interaction can be viewed as a result of a synthesis of the following functions: First, we have the capacity and extent of the network. Second, we have the conceivable topology of the network—that is, the way in which the aggregate of alternatives can be arranged. Third, we deal with the problems of predictability—that is, the information which a part possesses about the other part and about the whole system.

At the intrapersonal level, the capacity and the extent of the network are more or less known to a scientific observer, who may be the participant himself. At this level the possibilities of rearrangement are limited, and therefore the organism can somewhat predict its own reactions. At the interpersonal level, the capacity and extent of the network are still within assessable range. But because the topology of the interpersonal system is undefined, it is difficult if not impossible to predict future events within the realm of the system.

At the group level the extent of the network may be large, but inasmuch as there is a specialization of the functions of the interacting individuals, the behavior of the group as a whole becomes more predictable than the behavior of non-organized aggregates. It is, however, necessary to add that one effect of defining the function of the participating individuals is that the individuals themselves become less able to perceive the characteristics of the total group from within.

At the cultural level, the temporal and spatial limits of the network are not perceptible to the participants, who also are incapable of perceiving its topology. Therefore, for the participants, predictability is minimal and excessively difficult for the scientific observer.

At all levels, the degree of self-correction is a function of the entity's ability to predict (see ref. 134).

B. *Information and action.* In discussing information and the exchanges of information, it is necessary to insist upon a dual relationship between information and action. At one level it is true that goal-directed behavior is corrected by processes of feedback. At another level, it is necessary to recognize that action liberates codified information which is unavailable until the action is in full progress. This relation between practice and learning obtains not only at the intrapersonal level, but also at all other levels.

Destructive interaction, in which individuals move either towards self-destruction or towards breaking down the system in which they participate, may be due to several factors. First, such action may result from incomplete information about the self, the other persons, or the system. Second, there are the discrepancies in the evaluation of goals and instrumental actions; for example, a self-maximizing tendency (see p. 183) may lead to destruction of some larger system which was instrumental and necessary to the existence of the self. In special cases, the self-destruction of the smaller entity is instrumental to the survival of the larger system. The purpose of any action can, as of today, be discussed only after delineating the system to whose maintenance the action contributes. For such delineation an observer is necessary. The problems of purpose in cosmic and biological systems beyond the scope of our observation and comprehension cannot be meaningfully discussed.

REFERENCES

1. Alexander, F.: "The Logic of Emotions and Its Dynamic Background." *Int. J. of Psychoanalysis*, 16:399–413, 1935.

2. Alexander, F.: *Psychosomatic Medicine—Its Principles and Applications*. 320 pp. New York, Norton, 1950.

3. Alexander, F., and French, T. M.: *Psychoanalytic Therapy*. 353 pp. New York, Ronald Press, 1946.

4. Alexander, F., and French, T. M.: *Studies in Psychosomatic Medicine*. 568 pp. New York, Ronald Press, 1948.

5. Allen, F. H., Diethelm, O., and Sullivan, H. S.: "Report of Committee on Psychotherapy." *Amer. J. Psychiat.*, 101:266–267, 1944.

6. Allen, F. H.: *Psychotherapy with Children*. 311 pp. New York, Norton, 1942.

7. Allen, F. L.: *Only Yesterday*. 413 pp. New York, Harper & Bros., 1932.

8. Allport, G. W.: "The Ego in Contemporary Psychology." *Psychol. Rev.* 50:451–478, 1943.

9. Anderson, S.: *Winesburg, Ohio*. 303 pp. New York, Viking, 1919.

10. Baker, J.: Letter to *Look*, Vol. 13, No. 20, Sept. 27, 1949.

11. Balint, M.: "On the Psychoanalytic Training System," *Int. J. of Psychoanalysis*, 29:163–173, 1948.

12. Barker, R. G., Wright, B. A., and Gonick, M. R.: *Adjustment to Physical Handicap and Illness: A Survey of the Social Psychology of Physique and Disability*. 372 pp. New York, Soc. Sc. Res. Council Bull. 55, 1946.

13. Bateson, G.: "Culture Contact and Schismogenesis." *Man,* 35:178–183, 1935.

14. Bateson, G.: *Naven.* 286 pp. London, Cambridge Univ. Press, 1936.

15. Bateson, G.: "Experiments in Thinking about Observed Ethnological Material." *Philos. of Sc.,* 8:53–68, 1940.

16. Bateson, G.: "The Frustration-Aggression Hypothesis." *Psychol. Rev.,* 48:350–355, 1941.

17. Bateson, G.: "Regularities and Differences in National Character," in Watson, G., *Civilian Morale.* Boston, Houghton Mifflin, 1942.

18. Bateson, G.: *Social Planning and the Concept of "Deutero-Learning."* Conference on Science, Philosophy and Religion, Second Symposium. New York, Harper, 1942, pp. 81–97.

19. Bateson, G.: "The Science of Decency." *Phil. of Sc.,* 10:140–142, 1943.

20. Bateson, G.: "Cultural Determinants of Personality" in *Personality and the Behavior Disorders.* New York, Ronald, 1944, Vol. II, pp. 714–733.

21. Bateson, G.: "Bali: The Value System of a Steady State" in "Social Structure Studies," presented to A. R. Radcliffe-Brown. Oxford University Press, 1949, pp. 35–53.

22. Bateson, G., and Mead, M.: *Balinese Character, a Photographic Analysis.* 277 pp. New York, New York Acad. Sc., 1942.

23. Beard, C. A., and Beard, M. R.: *The Rise of American Civilization.* 2 vols. New York, Macmillan, 1937.

24. Beck, B. M., and Robbins, L. L.: *Short-Term Therapy in an Authoritative Setting.* 112 pp. New York, Family Service Association, 1946.

25. Benedict, R. F.: *Patterns of Culture.* 272 pp. Boston, Houghton Mifflin, 1934.

26. Bernard, C.: *Les phénomènes de la Vie.* 2 vols. Paris, 1878.

27. Berkeley, E.: *Giant Brains or Machines That Think.* 270 pp. New York, Wiley, 1949.

28. Bertalanffy, L. von: "The Theory of Open Systems in Physics and Biology." *Science,* 111:23–29, 1950.

29. Born, M.: *Natural Philosophy of Cause and Chance.* 215 pp. London, Oxford University Press, 1949.

30. Brenman, M., and Gill, M.: *Hypnotherapy—a Survey of Literature.* 276 pp. New York, Int. Univ. Press, 1947.

31. Brill, A. A.: "Various Schools of Psychotherapy." *Conn. St. Med. J.,* 7:530–536, 1943.

32. Brogan, D. W.: *The American Character.* 169 pp. New York, Knopf, 1944.

33. Brunswik, E.: "Points of View," in *Encyclopedia of Psychology.* New York, Philosophical Library, 1946, pp. 523–537.

34. Brunswik, E.: *Systematic and Representative Design of Psychological Experiments with Results in Physical and Social Perception.* Univ. of Calif. Syllabus Series, No. 304. Berkeley, Univ. of Calif. Press, 1947, p. 60.

35. Bush, V.: *Science the Endless Frontier.* 184 pp. Washington, U.S. Government Printing Office, 1945.

36. Cannon, W. B.: *Bodily Changes in Pain, Hunger, Fear and Rage.* 404 pp. New York, Appleton, 1929.

37. Cannon, W. B.: *The Wisdom of the Body.* 312 pp. New York, Norton, 1932.

38. Carnegie, D. C.: *How to Win Friends and Influence People.* 337 pp. New York, Simon and Schuster, 1936.

39. Cobb, S.: *Borderlands of Psychiatry.* 166 pp. Cambridge, Harvard University Press, 1943.

40. Cobb, S.: *Foundations of Neuropsychiatry.* 260 pp. Baltimore, Williams and Wilkins, 1948.

41. Collingwood, R. G.: *Principles of Art.* 360 pp. Oxford University Press, 1938.

42. Collingwood, R. G.: *The Idea of History.* 366 pp. Oxford University Press, 1946.

43. Collingwood, R. G.: *Speculum Mentis.* 328 pp. Oxford University Press, 1946.

44. Combs, A. W., Durkin, H. E., Hutt, M. L., Miller, J. G., Moreno, J. L., and Thorne, F. C.: "Current Trends in Clinical Psychology." *Ann. N.Y. Acad. Sc.,* 49:867–928, 1948.

45. Craik, K. J. W.: *The Nature of Explanation.* 123 pp. Cambridge University Press, 1943.

46. Davis, J. E.: *Principles and Practice of Recreational Therapy for the Mentally Ill.* 206 pp. New York, Barnes, 1936.

47. de Tocqueville, A.: *Democracy in America.* 2 vols. New York, Knopf, 1946.

48. Dollard, J., Doob, L. M., Miller, N. E., Mowrer, O. H., and Sears, R. R.: *Frustration and Aggression.* 209 pp. New Haven, Yale University Press, 1939.

49. Dos Passos, J.: *U.S.A.* 561 pp. New York, Modern Library, 1939.

50. Dunbar, F.: *Emotions and Bodily Changes. A Survey of Literature on Psychosomatic Interrelationships.* 1910–1945. 3rd ed. 604 pp. New York, Columbia University Press, 1946.

51. Dunbar, F.: *Synopsis of Psychosomatic Diagnosis and Treatment.* 501 pp. St. Louis, C. V. Mosby, 1948.

52. Erikson, E. H.: "Configurations in Play—Clinical Notes." *Psychoanal. Quart.,* 6:139–214, 1937.

53. Erikson, E. H.: "Ego Development and Historical Change. Clinical Notes." *Psychoanal. Study of the Child,* II, 359–396, 1946.

54. Fenichel, O.: *The Psychoanalytic Theory of Neurosis.* 703 pp. New York, Norton, 1945.

55. French, L. M.: *Psychiatric Social Work.* 344 pp. New York, Commonwealth Fund, 1940.

56. Fromm, E.: *Man for Himself: an Inquiry into the Psychology of Ethics.* 254 pp. New York, Rinehart, 1947.

57. Group for the Advancement of Psychiatry: Circular Letter No. 114, "Reports on Problems of Psychotherapy." 1948.

58. Gerard, R. W.: "A Biological Basis for Ethics." *Philos. of Sc.,* 9:92–120, 1942.

59. Ginsburg, S. W.: "Values and the Psychiatrist." *Am. J. Orthopsychiat.,* 20:466–478, 1950.

60. Glover, E., Fenichel, O., Strachey, J., Bergler, E., Nunberg, H., and Bibring, E.: "Symposium on the Theory of the Therapeutic Results of Psychoanalysis." *Int. J. Psychoanal.* 18:125–189, 1937.

61. Glover, E.: *Basic Mental Concepts, Their Clinical and Theoretical Value.* 32 pp. London, Imago Publishing Company, 1947.

62. Glueck, B.: *Current Therapies of Personality Disorders.* 296 pp. New York, Grune & Stratton, 1946.

63. Gödel, K.: "Über formal unentscheidbare Sätze der Principia Mathematica und verwandte Systeme." *Monatschr. Math. Phys.,* 38:173–198, 1931.

64. Goldstein, K.: *The Organism, a Holistic Approach to Biology.* 533 pp. New York, American Book Company, 1939.

65. Gorer, G.: *The American People.* 246 pp. New York, Norton, 1948.

66. Grinker, R. R., and Spiegel, J. P.: *Men under Stress.* 484 pp. Philadelphia, Blakiston, 1945.

67. Grinker, R. R., and Spiegel, J. P.: *War Neuroses.* 143 pp. Philadelphia, Blakiston, 1945.

68. *Group Psychotherapy: A Symposium.* 300 pp. New York, Beacon, 1945.

69. Gunther, J.: *Inside U.S.A.* 979 pp. New York, Harper, 1947.

70. Haas, L. J.: *Practical Occupational Therapy for the Mentally and Nervously Ill.* 432 pp. Milwaukee, Bruce, 1944.

71. Hamilton, G.: *Psychotherapy in Child Guidance.* 340 pp. New York, Columbia University Press, 1947.

72. Harlow, H. E.: "The Formation of Learning Sets." *Psychol. Rev.,* 56:51–65, 1949.

73. Hayakawa, S. I.: *Language in Thought and Action: a Guide to Accurate Thinking, Reading, and Writing.* 307 pp. New York, Harcourt Brace, 1949.

74. Hilgard, E. R., and Marquis, D. G.: *Conditioning and Learning.* 429 pp. New York, Appleton, 1940.

75. Hilgard, E. R.: *Theories of Learning.* 361 pp. New York, Appleton, 1948.

76. Horney, K.: *The Neurotic Personality of Our Time.* 299 pp. New York, Norton, 1937.

77. Horsley, J. S.: *Narco-Analysis.* 143 pp. London, Oxford University Press, 1943.

REFERENCES 295

78. Hubbard, L. R.: *Dianetics, the Modern Science of Mental Health.* 452 pp. New York, Hermitage, 1950.

79. Hull, E. L., and others: *Mathematico-Deductive Theory of Rote Learning.* 329 pp. Yale University, Institute of Human Relations, 1940.

80. Hutchinson, G. E.: Circular Causal Systems in Ecology. *Ann. of N.Y. Acad. of Sc.,* 50:221–246, 1948.

81. Jacobson, E.: *Progressive Relaxation.* 429 pp. Chicago, University of Chicago Press, 1929.

82. James, H.: *The American.* 540 pp. New York, Houghton Mifflin, 1877.

83. Janet, P.: *Principles of Psychotherapy.* 322 pp. New York, Macmillan, 1924.

84. Janet, P.: *Psychological Healing.* 2 vols. New York, Macmillan, 1925.

85. Kardiner, A.: *The Psychological Frontiers of Society.* 475 pp. New York, Columbia University Press, 1945.

86. Keyserling, H. A.: *America Set Free.* 609 pp. New York, Harper, 1929.

87. Kinsey, A. C., Pomeroy, W. B., and Martin, C. E.: *Sex Behavior in the Human' Male.* 804 pp. Philadelphia, Saunders, 1948.

88. Kluckhohn, C., and Kluckhohn, F. R.: "American Culture: Generalized Orientations and Class Patterns," in *Conflicts of Power in Modern Culture.* New York, Harper, 1947, pp. 106–128.

89. Köhler, W.: *Gestalt Psychology.* 369 pp. New York, Liveright, 1947.

90. Korzybski, A.: *Science and Sanity.* New York, Science Press, 1941.

91. Kraepelin, E.: *Clinical Psychiatry.* Adapted from the 6th German edition of Kraepelin's *Lehrbuch der Psychiatrie* by A. Ross Defendorf. 420 pp. New York, Macmillan, 1904.

92. Krech, D. C., and Crutchfield, R. S.: *Theory and Problems of Social Psychology.* 639 pp. New York, McGraw-Hill, 1948.

93. Kubie, L. S.: The Nature of Psychotherapy, *Bull. N.Y. Acad. Med.* 19:183–194, 1943.

94. Kubie, L. S.: "Fallacious Use of Quantitative Concepts in Dynamic Psychology." *Psychoanal. Quart.*, 16:507–518, 1947.

95. Laski, H. J.: *The American Democracy.* 785 pp. New York, Viking, 1948.

96. Lee, D.: "Lineal and Non-Lineal Codification of Reality." *Psychosom. Med.*, 12:89–97, 1950.

97. Lewin, R.: A *Dynamic Theory of Personality.* 286 pp. New York, McGraw-Hill, 1935.

98. Lewis, S.: *Babbitt.* 401 pp. New York, Harcourt, 1922.

99. Licht, S.: *Music in Medicine.* 132 pp. Boston, New England Conservatory of Music, 1946.

100. Liddell, H. S.: "Reflex Method and Experimental Neurosis," in *Personality and the Behavior Disorders.* New York, Ronald Press, 1944, pp. 389–412.

101. Lief, A.: *The Common-Sense Psychiatry of Dr. Adolph Meyer.* 677 pp. New York, McGraw-Hill, 1948.

102. Linklater, E.: *Don Juan in America.* 466 pp. New York, Farrar, 1931.

103. Lippitt, R.: "An Experimental Study of the Effect of Democratic and Authoritarian Group Atmospheres." *Univ. Iowa Stud. Child Welf.*, 16:43–195, 1940.

104. Lowrey, L. G.: "Trends in Orthopsychiatric Therapy: General Developments and Trends." *Am. J. Orthopsychiat.*, 18:381–394, 1948.

105. McCulloch, W. S., and Pitts, W.: "A Logical Calculus of the Ideas Immanent in Nervous Activity." *Bull. of Math. Biophys.*, 5:115–133, 1943.

106. McCulloch, W. S.: "A Heterarchy of Values, Etc." *Bull. of Math. Biophys.*, 7:89–93, 1945.

107. McCulloch, W. S.: "A Recapitulation of the Theory, with a Forecast of Several Extensions." *Ann. of N.Y. Acad. Sc.*, 50:259–277, 1948.

108. McCulloch, W. S., and Pitts, W.: "How We Recognize Universals." *Bull. of Math. Biophys.* 1947.

109. Madariaga, S. de: *Englishmen, Frenchmen, Spaniards.* 256 pp. London, Oxford University Press, 1928.

110. Mannheim, K.: *Ideology and Utopia.* 318 pp. New York, Harcourt Brace, 1949.

111. Mannheim, K.: *Man and Society in an Age of Reconstruction.* 469 pp. New York, Harcourt Brace, 1949.

112. Mead, M.: *And Keep Your Powder Dry.* 274 pp. New York, Morrow, 1942.

113. Mead, M.: *Sex and Temperament in Three Primitive Societies.* New York, Morrow, 1935.

114. Miller, N. E., and Dollard, J.: *Social Learning and Imitation.* 341 pp. New Haven, Yale University Press, 1941.

115. Moreno, J. L.: *Psychodrama.* 429 pp. New York, Beacon, 1946.

116. Moreno, J. L.: "Contributions of Sociometry to Research Methodology in Sociology." *Am. Soc. Rev.,* 12:287–292, 1947.

117. Morris, C. W.: *Signs, Language and Behavior.* 365 pp. New York, Prentice-Hall, 1946.

118. Moulton, F., and others: *Mental Health.* 470 pp. Washington, Science Press, 1939.

119. Mowrer, O. H.: "Learning Theory and the Neurotic Paradox." *Am. J. Orthopsychiat.,* 18:571–610, 1948.

120. Mullahy, P., and others: *A Study of Interpersonal Relationships.* 507 pp. New York, Hermitage, 1949.

121. Murphy, G.: *Historical Introduction to Modern Psychology.* 466 pp. New York, Harcourt Brace, 1949.

122. Nicole, J. E.: *Psychopathology—A Survey of Modern Approaches.* 4th ed. 268 pp. Baltimore, Williams and Wilkins, 1947.

123. Oberndorf, C. P.: "Constant Elements in Psychotherapy." *Psychoanal. Quart.,* 15:435–449, 1946.

124. Ogden, C. K., and Richards, I. A.: *The Meaning of Meaning.* 363 pp. New York, Routledge, 1936.

125. *One Hundred Years of American Psychiatry.* 649 pp. New York, Columbia University Press, 1944.

126. Parrington, V. L.: *Main Currents in American Thought*. 3 vols. New York, Harcourt Brace, 1927.

127. Parsons, T.: *Essays in Sociological Theory, Pure and Applied*. 366 pp. Glencoe, Illinois, Free Press, 1949.

128. Pavlov, I. P.: *Lectures on Conditioned Reflexes*. 414 pp. New York, Int. Publishers, 1928.

129. Rennie, T. A. C., and Woodward, L. E.: *Mental Health in Modern Society*. 424 pp. New York, Commonwealth Fund, 1948.

130. Riesman, D.: "Authority and Liberty in the Structure of Freud's Thought." *Psychiatry*, 13:167–187, 1950.

131. Riesman, D.: "The Themes of Work and Play in the Structure of Freud's Thought." *Psychiatry*, 13:1–16, 1950.

132. Roethlisberger, F. J.: *Management and Morale*. 194 pp. Cambridge, Harvard University Press, 1949.

133. Rogers, C. R.: *Counseling and Psychotherapy*. 450 pp. New York, Houghton Mifflin, 1942.

134. Rosenblueth, A., Wiener, N., and Bigelow, J.: "Behavior, Purpose, and Teleology." *J. Philos. Sc.*, 10:18–24, 1943.

135. Ruesch, J., Harris, R. E., Loeb, M. B., Christiansen, C., Dewees, M. S., Heller, S. H., and Jacobson, A.: *Chronic Disease and Psychological Invalidism—A Psychosomatic Study*. 191 pp. New York, Am. Soc. Res. Psychosom. Probl., 1946.

136. Ruesch, J., Christiansen, C., Patterson, L. C., Dewees, S., and Jacobson, A.: "Psychological Invalidism in Thyroidectomized Patients." *Psychosom. Med.* 9:77–91, 1947.

137. Ruesch, J.: "What Are the Known Facts about Psychosomatic Medicine at the Present Time?" *J. Soc. Case W.*, 28:291–296, 1947.

138. Ruesch, J.: "Experiments in Psychotherapy: 1. Theoretical Considerations." *J. Psych.*, 28:137–169, 1948.

139. Ruesch, J., and Bowman, K. M.: "Personality and Chronic Illness." *J.A.M.A.*, 136:851–855, 1948.

140. Ruesch, J.: "Social Technique, Social Status and Social Change in Illness," in *Personality in Nature, Society and Culture*. New York, Knopf, 1948, pp. 117–130.

141. Ruesch, J.: "The Infantile Personality: The Core Problem of Psychosomatic Medicine." *Psychosom. Med.*, 3:134–144, 1948.

142. Ruesch, J., Harris, R. E., Christiansen, C., Loeb, M. B., Dewees, S., and Jacobson, A.: *Duodenal Ulcer—A Socio-psychological Study of Naval Enlisted Personnel and Civilians.* 118 pp. Berkeley and Los Angeles, University of California Press, 1948.

143. Ruesch, J., Jacobson, A., and Loeb, M. B.: *Acculturation and Illness.* 40 pp. Psych. Mon. Gen. Appl., 62, No. 5, 1948.

144. Ruesch, J.: "An Investigation of Prediction of Success in Naval Flight Training. Psychological Tests." Pp. 115–152 in Report No. 81, and pp. 65–83 in Report No. 82. Washington, Civil Aeronautics Administration, 1948.

145. Ruesch, J.: "Individual Social Techniques." *J. Soc. Psychol.*, 29:3–28, 1949.

146. Ruesch, J.: "Mastery of Long-Term Illness," in *Medical Clinics of North America.* Philadelphia, Saunders, 1949, pp. 435–446.

147. Ruesch, J., and Bateson, G.: "Structure and Process in Social Relations." *Psychiatry*, 12:105–124, 1949.

148. Ruesch, J., and Prestwood, A. R.: "Anxiety: Its Initiation, Communication and Interpersonal Management." *Arch. Neurol. & Psychiat.*, 62:527–550, 1949.

149. Ruesch, J., and Prestwood, A. R.: "Interaction Processes and Personal Codification." *J. Personality*, 18:391–430, 1950.

150. Ruesch, J., and Prestwood, A. R.: "Communication and Bodily Disease," in *Life Stress and Bodily Disease.* Assoc. Res. Nerv. Ment. Dis., 29:211–230, 1950.

151. Ruesch, J.: "Part and Whole," *Dialectica.* Vol. 4, No. 3, 1950.

152. Sapir, E.: "Communication." *Encyc. Soc. Sc.*, 1931, Vol. 4, pp. 78–80.

153. Schrödinger, E.: *What Is Life?* 91 pp. New York, Macmillan, 1946.

154. Selling, L. S., and Ferraro, M. A.: *The Psychology of Diet and Nutrition.* 192 pp. New York, Norton, 1945.

155. Shannon, C. E., and Weaver, W.: *The Mathematical Theory*

of Communication. 116 pp. Urbana, University of Illinois Press, 1949.

156. Shaw, R. F.: *Fingerpainting.* 232 pp. Boston, Little, Brown, 1938.

157. Siegfried, A.: *Les Etats-Unis d'aujourd'hui.* 362 pp. Paris, Armand Colin, 1939.

158. Spengler, O.: *Der Untergang des Abendlandes.* 2 vols. Munich, Beck, 1923.

159. Strachey, J.: "The Nature of the Therapeutic Action of Psychoanalysis." *Int. J. Psychoanal.,* 15:127–159, 1934.

160. Sullivan, H. S.: "Conceptions of Modern Psychiatry." *Psychiatry,* 3:1–117, 1940.

161. Szurek, S.: "Emotional Factors in the Use of Authority," in *Public Health Is People.* New York, Commonwealth Fund, 1950, pp. 222–225.

162. Taft, D. R.: *Criminology.* 708 pp. New York, Macmillan, 1943.

163. Thompson, C.: *Psychoanalysis: Evolution and Development.* 250 pp. New York, Hermitage, 1950.

164. Tinbergen, N.: *Objectivistic Study of the Innate Behavior of Animals.* 64 pp. Bibliotheca Biotheoretica. New York, Brill, 1942.

165. Titchener, E. B.: *Experimental Psychology.* 2 vols. New York, Macmillan, 1910.

166. Toynbee, A. J.: *A Study of History.* 617 pp. New York, Oxford University Press, 1947.

167. Trollope, A.: *North America.* 2 vols. London, Chapman and Hall, 1862.

168. Von Neumann, J., and Morgenstern, O.: *Theory of Games and Economic Behavior.* 625 pp. Princeton University Press, 1944.

169. Wach, J.: *Das Verstehen—Grundzüge einer Geschichte der hermeneutischen Theorie im 19. Jahrhundert.* 3 vols. Tübingen, Mohr, 1926–1933.

170. Warner, W. L., Meeker, M., and Eells, K.: *Social Class in America.* 274 pp. Chicago, Science Res. Association, 1949.

171. Watson, J. B.: *Behaviorism.* Revised ed. 308 pp. New York, Norton, 1930.

172. Weber, M.: *The Protestant Ethic and the Spirit of Capitalism.* 292 pp. London, Allen and Unwin, 1930.

173. Weigert, E.: "Existentialism and Its Relation to Psychotherapy," *Psychiatry,* 12:399–412, 1949.

174. Weiss, E., and English, O. S.: *Psychosomatic Medicine.* 687 pp. Philadelphia, Saunders, 1943.

175. West, J.: *Plainville, U.S.A.* 238 pp. New York, Columbia University Press, 1945.

176. Weyl, H.: *Philosophy of Mathematics and Natural Science.* 311 pp. Princeton University Press, 1944.

177. Whitehead, A. N., and Russell, B.: *Principia Mathematica.* 3 vols. 2nd ed. Cambridge, 1910–13.

178. Whitehead, A. N.: *Symbolism, Its Meaning and Effects.* 88 pp. New York, Macmillan, 1927.

179. Whyte, L. L.: *The Unitary Principle in Physics and Biology.* 163 pp. New York, Holt, 1949.

180. Wiener, N.: *Cybernetics or Control and Communication in the Animal and the Machine.* 194 pp. New York, Wiley, 1948.

181. Wiener, N.: *The Human Use of Human Beings—Cybernetics and Society.* 241 pp. Boston, Houghton Mifflin, 1950.

182. Wittgenstein, L.: *Tractatus Logico-Philosophicus.* 189 pp. London, Harcourt Brace, 1922.

183. Wolberg, L. R.: *Medical Hypnosis.* 2 vols. New York, Grune and Stratton, 1948.

184. Whorf, B. L.: "Science and Linguistics." *Technology Rev.,* 44:229–248, 1940.

185. Wundt, W.: *Principles of Physiological Psychology.* 2 vols. New York, Macmillan, 1873–1874.

186. Zilboorg, G.: *A History of Medical Psychology.* 606 pp. New York, Norton, 1941.

187. Zipf, G. K.: *Human Behavior and the Principle of Least Effort.* 573 pp. Cambridge, Addison-Wesley, 1949.

INDEX

Printed in the United States
by Baker & Taylor Publisher Services

Printed in the United States
by Baker & Taylor Publisher Services